# Fuel for Young Athletes

Ann Litt, MS, RD

# Fuel for Young Athletes

Ann Litt, MS, RD

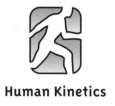

**Human Kinetics**

Library of Congress Cataloging-in-Publication Data

Litt, Ann, 1953-
  Fuel for young athletes / Ann Litt.
    p. cm.
Includes index.
  ISBN 0-7360-4652-6 (soft cover)
  1. High school athletes--Nutrition. 2. Child athletes--Nutrition. I.
Title.
  TX361.A8L52 2003
  613.2'024'796--dc21                                    2003008764

ISBN-10: 0-7360-4652-6
ISBN-13: 978-0-7360-4652-7

The Web addresses cited in this text were current as of August 2003, unless otherwise noted.

**Developmental Editor:** Laura Hambly; **Assistant Editors:** Alisha Jeddeloh and Anna FitzSimmons; **Copyeditor:** John Wentworth; **Proofreader:** Jim Burns; **Indexer:** Bobbi Swanson; **Permission Manager:** Toni Harte; **Graphic Designer:** Andrew Tietz; **Graphic Artist:** Kim McFarland; **Art and Photo Manager:** Dan Wendt; **Cover Designer:** Kristin A. Darling; **Photographer (cover):** Tom Roberts; **Photographer (interior):** © Human Kinetics; **Illustrators:** Roberto Sabas (graphs) and Dick Flood (drawing on page 52); **Printer:** United Graphics

Human Kinetics books are available at special discounts for bulk purchase. Special editions or book excerpts can also be created to specification. For details, contact the Special Sales Manager at Human Kinetics.

Printed in the United States of America          10  9  8

The paper in this book is certified under a sustainable forestry program.

**Human Kinetics**
Web site: www.HumanKinetics.com

*United States:* Human Kinetics
P.O. Box 5076
Champaign, IL 61825-5076
800-747-4457
e-mail: humank@hkusa.com

*Canada:* Human Kinetics
475 Devonshire Road, Unit 100
Windsor, ON N8Y 2L5
800-465-7301 (in Canada only)
e-mail: info@hkcanada.com

*Europe:* Human Kinetics
107 Bradford Road
Stanningley
Leeds LS28 6AT, United Kingdom
+44 (0)113  255  5665
e-mail: hk@hkeurope.com

*Australia:* Human Kinetics
57A Price Avenue
Lower Mitcham, South Australia 5062
08 8372 0999
e-mail: info@hkaustralia.com

*New Zealand:* Human Kinetics
P.O. Box 80
Torrens Park, South Australia 5062
0800 222 062
e-mail: info@hknewzealand.com

To MY4SOME—Dan, David, and Jordan,
who support and encourage me in every way possible

# Contents

# Preface

When I was a competitive swimmer, from 1961 to 1968, we knew nothing about the importance of nutrition for athletes. Like all young athletes, I would have done anything to be a faster swimmer. My coach was my only source of information, and I hung on to each bit of advice he offered. It was just my luck that my coach believed oranges were better to eat than candy. Perhaps that had something to do with my appreciation for eating well.

We've come a long way since then. Sports nutrition was born, and with our new knowledge about how to improve performance through training and eating properly, athletes are now smashing records like never before.

Feeding growing athletes is serious work. Facing you are the challenges of ensuring your athletes are getting enough nutrients for growth; teaching them the right mixes of foods to optimize performance and when to eat them; and dealing with the quirkiness of the young, undeveloped palate. You'll need to learn to work around haphazard training schedules that interfere with normal meal times, peer pressure young athletes face to skip meals, and of course fast food and vending machines positioned at every turn. Today, when it's so easy to grab whatever food is there that fills you up so you can get going again, there's more need than ever to make sure young athletes learn the basics about nutrition and eating right.

You'll want to be aware of what influences and motivates teenagers. Young athletes look to their college and professional counterparts as role models. They'll be tempted to use some of the techniques, supplements, and regimens used and promoted by older athletes. When it comes to how our young athletes train and feed their bodies, we need to help them understand that they are still growing and that what might be appropriate for a college or professional athlete might not be best for them.

While most young athletes demonstrate an extraordinary degree of discipline and are eager to do whatever it takes to improve their performance, they are still teenagers. They'll be tempted to use supplements, take shortcuts, and pursue risks. We should not dismiss their decisions or be judgmental but rather work with them, using their many concerns and questions as springboards for discussion.

We have lofty goals for nourishing young athletes. We want them to grow to their full potential. We want them to eat a diet that's both good for long-term health and gives them a competitive edge. One point I'll reiterate in this book is that young athletes are neither interested in nor motivated by information about food's role in promoting good health. You'll reach them best by showing them how eating right can help them right now. Once they experience for themselves how adequate hydration helps them through a workout, how eating breakfast makes them less tired, and how a postwork-out snack helps them recover from training, they're on their way toward a new respect for nutrition and the benefits of eating right.

As the parent of two former high school athletes, I have lived the hectic pace experienced by families of athletes. Putting sports nutrition into practice takes time. Convenience, taste, and cost often influence what we choose to feed our young athletes. It takes effort and commitment to drive past the local McDonald's toward a better meal down the road.

As a sports nutritionist, my expertise is boiling down the science of nutrition into the art of making the information useful. I have found that if you can communicate the right message in a teenager-friendly way, your young athletes will use and appreciate your guidance. You can be instrumental in teaching the lifelong lessons that come from eating well. Eating for sport works, and *Fuel for Young Athletes* can help you put a plan in place. Your young athletes will feel great and get the results they're looking for through proper training and learning to eat like an athlete.

# Acknowledgments

Writing a book provides the pleasure of publicly thanking those who help you, even when they may not realize it. My thanks go to . . .

all of the parents and coaches who gave me access to their athletes;

the wonderful athletes who allowed me to help them change their diets, shared with me team dynamics, and sometimes ate in my kitchen;

my incredible nutrition colleagues, especially Nancy Clark, who turned me on to this project;

my terrific friends, who always made sure I didn't become a recluse while writing by scheduling lunches and helping me stay active;

my editor at Human Kinetics, Laura Hambly, who coached me through this project and stuck with me throughout; and

MY4SOME—my family of golfers, who have learned how to enjoy good food on and off the course but, more important, have learned so many life lessons through sports.

Finally, thanks to my parents, who encouraged me to be an athlete before it was a matter of course for girls to compete and long before the benefits of Title IX.

# Chapter 1

# FOOD FUNCTIONS FOR DEVELOPING ATHLETES

Young athletes require high-quality fuel . . . and a lot of it. Children generally have a wide margin of error when it comes to eating a healthy diet, but the bodies of growing athletes are like expensive race cars: The better the fuel, the smoother the engine will run.

For young athletes to grow properly, play seriously, and stay healthy, they need to eat the right food in the correct amounts. If they don't, their bodies won't perform for them—they will have less energy than their peers, they will be more likely to get sick, and their training will be inadequate. Parents and coaches can help their young athletes understand that eating right directly affects training and competition. It is up to parents to provide nutritious meals and snacks and ensure that their busy children take time to eat well. Eating properly for their sport is as important as practicing the skills their sport requires. Coaches and parents have a wonderful opportunity to teach children the value of eating a healthy diet to help them perform better, grow properly, and stay healthy.

## The Fuel to Move

Food supplies us with fuel, otherwise known as calories. The body, regardless of age, gender, or activity level, burns a certain amount of calories just to stay alive. Calories are burned during normal body functions, such as pumping blood, breathing, and even batting eyelashes. The calories burned during these basic functions determine a body's *resting metabolic rate* (RMR). The RMR is simply the number of calories burned by the body to keep it going.

The amount of calories a particular body needs is influenced by many factors. Basic calorie ranges, which take into consideration the RMR, have been established for growing children (table 1.1). These ranges are just starting points for determining calorie needs and should be used only as a guide to get a general idea of the calories burned by active, growing children.

TABLE 1.1  Average Daily Calorie Intakes for Children

| Age | Male | Female |
|-----|------|--------|
| 11-14 | 2,500 | 2,200 |
| 15-18 | 3,000 | 2,200 |

Along with the basic calories athletes burn to run their bodies, they also burn calories through exercise. The longer and harder they exercise, the more calories they burn. We have well-documented formulas to determine how many calories an adult athlete burns playing various sports. These formulas, however, are not applicable to children. The formulas generally underestimate calories burned by child athletes by as much as 30 percent.

An adapted formula is included to help you determine a general range of the number of calories children burn while playing selected sports (table 1.2). To determine an estimate of the total calories expended, add the number of calories burned by playing the sport to the number of basic calories needed to run the body (table 1.3).

Setting an ideal calorie level for a growing athlete is tricky. The calories derived from written formulas and the average intake set for children and teenagers provide only a ballpark figure. Calorie needs fluctuate tremendously from child to child, depending on growth, age, and activity. To assign

TABLE 1.2  Average Calories Expended by Children Engaged in Various Sports (per 10 Minutes of Activity)

| Activity | Body weight in kg* | | | | | | | | | |
|----------|-----|-----|-----|-----|-----|-----|-----|-----|-----|-----|
|          | 20 | 25 | 30 | 35 | 40 | 45 | 50 | 55 | 60 | 65 |
| Basketball | 34 | 43 | 51 | 60 | 68 | 77 | 85 | 94 | 102 | 110 |
| Ice hockey | 52 | 65 | 78 | 91 | 104 | 117 | 130 | 143 | 156 | 168 |
| Running | 37 | 45 | 52 | 60 | 66 | 72 | 78 | 84 | 90 | 95 |
| Soccer | 36 | 45 | 54 | 63 | 72 | 81 | 90 | 99 | 108 | 117 |
| Swimming  (30 m/min.) | | | | | | | | | | |
| Breaststroke | 19 | 24 | 29 | 34 | 38 | 43 | 48 | 53 | 58 | 62 |
| Crawl | 25 | 31 | 37 | 43 | 49 | 56 | 62 | 68 | 74 | 80 |
| Back | 17 | 21 | 25 | 30 | 34 | 38 | 42 | 47 | 51 | 55 |

*To determine weight in kg, divide weight in pounds by 2.2.

Data from Bar-Or, O., 1983, *Pediatric Sports Medicine*, (New York, NY: Springer-Verlag).

**TABLE 1.3**     How Much Does Your Athlete Burn?

To determine the calories burned by a 120-pound 15-year-old female soccer player on a day she has a soccer game:

**Daily needs = X**

A 15-year-old female needs approximately 2,200 cal/day.

**Calories burned = Y**

Determine weight in kg: 120 ÷ 2.2 = 54.5 kg

60 minutes playing ÷ 10 = 6 x 99 = 594 calories / 60 minutes of activity

A 120-pound soccer player burns approximately 594 calories per hour.

**Total calories needed = X + Y**

2,200 + 594 = **2,794 calories needed on game day**

a specific calorie level is fruitless and ignores a child's innate capability to self-regulate his intake. Use tables 1.1, 1.2, and 1.3 only as tools to identify a general range of caloric needs, not to determine the caloric adequacy of a particular child's diet.

The best way to judge whether children are eating enough is to watch their growth and weight. Are they growing at the rate they should? Are they maintaining a good weight? "Enough" isn't necessarily what we think it should be. Enough means children are eating a healthy diet that gives them the energy they need to play, grow, and stay healthy. Although some adults are tempted to be very scientific in their approach, in this case practicality should prevail. Watch your athlete's energy level, weight, growth pattern, and general health. If these show the right measures, your athlete is probably eating enough calories.

When athletes don't eat enough food, their bodies protect themselves by slowing down their metabolism. A slow metabolism affects how athletes feel and perform. These athletes tire more easily, and their bodies lack the energy to grow as they should.

It is sometimes difficult for active, growing kids to keep up with the amount of food they need to eat. The adults in their lives need to be involved with their meal and snack planning. As an adult, make sure your young athlete eats and drinks properly before, during, and after practices and competitions. This helps athletes stay nourished and demonstrates a commitment to team nutrition.

# Growth and Performance

Each child grows at his or her own pace. If you want a sense of what "normal" growth means, look at a group of 13-year-old boys. You'll see quite a range of body shapes and sizes, and all of them are normal. Kids can be ultrasensitive about their changing bodies. As a coach, remember that well-intentioned comments about their changing bodies might be misunderstood or misinterpreted. If you're concerned about an athlete's food intake and how it might be affecting performance, speak with the athlete privately, never in front of teammates.

Coaches and parents need to be aware of body changes that occur in athletes as they grow. Try not to compare body size or food intake among individual athletes. Their changing bodies will affect how they play and how they feel. For instance, a female basketball player might get recognition for her height, but she might feel that she's very different from her peer group who has not yet grown, which could affect her self-esteem. The middle-school football player might think his big body is helpful on the field, but off the field he might be embarrassed by his extra fat.

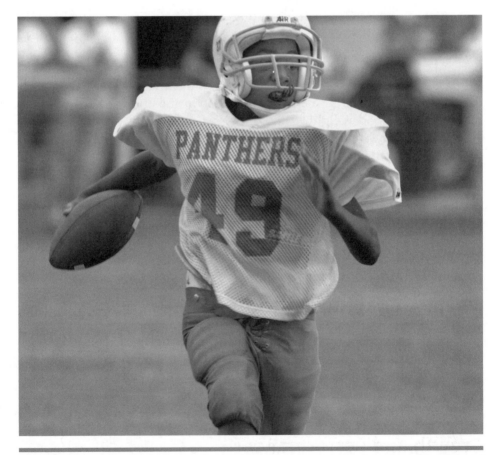

Young male athletes who develop later than their peers often become discouraged while waiting for strength to catch up with skill. Focusing on other areas, like good nutrition, is imperative.

Teenage girls, regardless of their sport, commonly want to be lean and fast. The prepubescent female athlete will need to lay down body fat to promote growth and allow for menstruation. Children living in our fat-phobic culture might be alarmed when fat becomes obvious on their bodies. Coaches and parents will surely notice the changing bodies of prepubescent girls. While too much fat might hamper performance and in some sports be undesirable, for the growing female athlete acquiring fat is just a developmental phase and needs to be appreciated. (See chapter 13 for a detailed discussion of this.) Helping your young athlete understand and accept her new body is an important part of your job.

Young male athletes present other challenges. They often focus on being stronger, bigger, and faster. Many late bloomers are discouraged when their bodies don't keep up with the growth of their peers, particularly when this affects their performance compared to that of their teammates. If the growth of late bloomers is assessed as being normal but on a slower than predicted curve, it is imperative that these children continue to fuel their bodies in a healthy way. Late bloomers are often discouraged; many drop out of their sport by the age of 13 because they don't allow for strength to catch up with skill. Parents and coaches can boost the confidence levels of these athletes by helping them develop in other important areas of their sport, such as speed, conditioning, and concentration. Pitchers might focus on control rather than on the speed of their fastball. Batters might work on increasing their batting average rather than trying to bang out homers before their body is ready.

Although we want them to be the best they can be in their sport, young athletes are still children and will be tempted to eat foods that aren't the best choices for them. Yes, help them be conscious of what they are putting into their bodies, but don't demand too much of them. The perfect diet for a growing athlete is all about balance. Young athletes need to know more than other children know about how food affects performance, but there's still room for less-than-perfect food choices within a good diet.

## Sleep: A Vital Nutrient

Using nutrients properly depends on getting enough rest. For an athlete, "rest" often means taking days off during training. Although this is important, our message here to teenagers is that they need to be mindful of the amount of sleep they get. Most teenagers are chronically sleep deprived. But to get the most out of nutrients, we need sleep to allow muscles to develop.

Sleep is key to performance. A well-rested athlete is more focused and less likely to make mental errors. While little research is available on how sleep affects nutrients and metabolism, at least one study on adults shows that sleep deprivation interferes with glucose metabolism, which affects endurance. Most parents recognize when their children are sleep deprived by watching them and noticing their energy levels. See table 1.4 for general guidelines on sleep requirements for adolescents. Connecting the importance of sleep to performance and to the body's proper use of nutrients makes for a more meaningful message to a teenage athlete.

TABLE 1.4    Sleep Guidelines

| Age | Total sleep hours needed |
| --- | --- |
| 7-9 years | 9.5-10.75 |
| 10-13 years | 9-10.5 |
| 14-18 years | 8.5-9.75 |

Data from *The Children's Hospital Guide to Your Child's Health and Development*, 2001, (Boulder, CO: Perseus Publication).

## Talking to Your Athlete About Food Functions

- Athletes have higher calorie needs than their nonathletic peers. We can estimate how much they need to eat, but the best indicator is how they grow and feel.
- Young athletes need to eat enough food to be healthy, support their activity, and grow.
- Athletes should power their bodies with the best fuel.
- All children grow at their own rate; growth and activity determine how much food a child needs. Discourage athletes from comparing their diets with others.
- Adequate sleep allows the body to use nutrients properly.

# Chapter 2

# NUTRITION ESSENTIALS FOR SPORTS

What makes a young athlete run fast, long, and injury free? A good training program, a driven athlete, and the right food. Young athletes perform better and feel better if they learn what, when, and how much to eat. They need to know what foods are important for energy, when to eat certain foods, how to eat during an event, and how to replenish their bodies so they can get out and do it again. All this is a tall order for kids who just want to eat.

When children eat, they don't really stop to consider whether the food is a good source of protein, fat, or carbohydrate. They eat because they are hungry; they eat what they like and avoid what they don't like. Kids can get by eating like kids. But growing athletes are different. Young athletes have the same nutritional needs as anyone else their age—they just need more. More food, more vitamins and minerals, and more fluids. Where they differ from other children is that they need to pay attention to their diets to ensure they have energy for practice, know the right foods to eat before a game, and drink plenty of fluids to stay well hydrated.

## Diet Basics

Food is a mixture of nutrients. Each nutrient has a specific job in nourishing the body. They are like team members, each with a role on the team. Some roles seem bigger than others, but no one nutrient is more important than another. They all must function in their role to get the job done.

The key nutrients found in food are protein, carbohydrates, fat, vitamins, minerals, and water. Of course, different foods supply different combinations of these nutrients. Protein, carbohydrates and fat—called *macronutrients*—supply the body with calories, which is the energy bodies use for fuel (table

**TABLE 2.1    Energy-Yielding Nutrients**

| |
|---|
| 1 gram of carbohydrates = 4 calories |
| 1 gram of protein = 4 calories |
| 1 gram of fat = 9 calories |
| 1 gram of alcohol = 7 calories |

2.1). Athletes need to know how they are fueling their bodies. They should understand what carbohydrates do for their energy level, how much protein they need, and how to consume the right amount of fat.

Vitamins and minerals are considered *micronutrients* because we need them in small amounts. They do not supply calories but are needed by the body to process food into energy. They help the body use calories and contribute vital, specific functions. Athletes require more vitamins and minerals than nonathletes do, but by eating more and choosing the right food athletes can easily get all of the extra vitamins and minerals they need. Rarely does an athlete need to take a vitamin-mineral supplement, although certain situations might require doing so. For instance, an athlete who cannot tolerate dairy might need a calcium supplement, or a strict vegetarian might need a vitamin $B_{12}$ supplement.

Water is a vital nutrient, too. Water is essential for everyone, but for athletes adequate hydration can make a big difference in how they feel, how they train, and how they perform. Water does not contribute calories to the diet, but without it we couldn't live.

## Carbohydrates: The All-Purpose Fuel

At least 50 percent of the calories an athlete eats should be from carbohydrates. This is the fuel muscles prefer for energy. All carbohydrates are converted to glucose to be used for energy. Carbohydrates produce four calories per gram when burned and are key ingredients before, during, and after exercising.

Different types of carbohydrates are found in food. Carbohydrates are classified as simple or complex, depending on how many units of glucose are linked together. *Simple* carbohydrates are one or two units of glucose, or sugar, linked together. They are found in foods that taste sweet, such as fruit, candy, cookies, and soft drinks. Simple carbohydrates are digested and absorbed quickly, so they are good sources for immediate fuel.

Eating a diet full of sweet-tasting carbohydrates (also known as "empty calories") affects energy level. Although simple carbohydrates tend to be in foods that taste good, they won't do anything for sustaining energy. Without a balance of other nutrients, an athlete attempting to subsist on simple carbohydrates will feel wiped out during training and competition.

*Complex* carbohydrates, sometimes called starch, are found in cereals, rice, potatoes, pasta, bread, beans, and some vegetables. Complex carbohydrates provide the body with calories as well as large amounts of vitamins, minerals, and fiber. Complex carbohydrates are digested and absorbed a bit slower

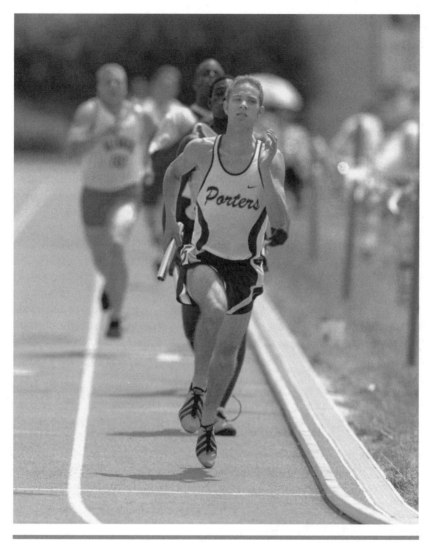

Carbohydrates provide the fuel an athlete needs to finish the race.

than simple carbohydrates and thus provide a longer lasting type of energy as well as many essential nutrients.

Carbohydrates are the primary fuel the body uses for energy. When glucose is not used immediately for energy, it is converted to glycogen that is stored in the muscles and the liver. Stored carbohydrates, or glycogen, are the most valuable and important fuel source for any athlete. Glycogen is the fuel that allows athletes to keep going. Training and diet influence the amount of glycogen an athlete can store in the muscles (see chapter 5). Carbohydrates that aren't burned for energy or converted to glycogen are stored by the body as fat.

All types of carbohydrates are important fuel. Complex carbohydrates with their package of important nutrients should provide the majority of carbohydrates consumed, but some simple carbohydrates are fine in an otherwise healthy diet.

## Alcohol and Teens

Underage drinking is a real problem for today's teenagers. According to one survey, 87 percent of high school seniors admitted to trying alcohol during high school. In fact, research reports that high school seniors consume their first alcoholic beverage at the average age of 14 years old. Giving young athletes the facts on how alcohol interferes with performance is one way to discourage underage drinking.

Alcoholic beverages are high in calories—seven calories a gram—but these calories are not used for energy by the body in the same way protein, carbohydrates, and fat are used. Alcohol can interfere with normal metabolism of these nutrients as well as with how the body uses vitamins and minerals. Furthermore, typical food choices while under the influence of alcohol are generally poor sources of nutrients and high in fat.

Although some teenagers say they feel more alert after drinking alcohol, in reality alcohol negatively affects coordination, judgment, and all aspects of performance. Alcohol intake also disrupts temperature regulation and fluid balance. The effects of alcohol consumption often carry over to the next day. Trying to compete or train with a hangover is not productive or enjoyable. Because teenagers tend to feel invincible, they rarely think beyond the next day, so adults need to stress to their young athletes the destructive powers of alcohol on the body. Long-term effects include liver damage, increased risk of developing certain cancers, and an increase in mortality. Help them understand this, but also emphasize that drinking alcohol makes it tougher for them to achieve their goals on the court or playing field. If you remind them how much ground a drinking athlete loses to a nondrinking athlete, your serious young athletes will listen closely.

### Protein: For Muscles and More

Because it is involved in building muscle and repairing muscle tissue after injury or exercise, protein is important to athletes. It is a part of all cells, including hair, skin, tissue, and muscles. Protein regulates body functions and keeps the body healthy and strong by fighting infections. Athletes, especially growing athletes, need more protein than nonathletes. Even though it is extremely important, it accounts for only about 20 percent of the calories in the diet. It is possible for young athletes to get plenty of protein by eating a balanced diet.

Protein is made up of small building blocks called amino acids. The body uses 20 amino acids that are linked together in varying sequences to form different types of protein needed by the body. Of the 20 amino acids the body requires, the body can make 11 on its own. These are called nonessential amino acids. The remaining 9 amino acids are called essential amino acids because the body cannot make them and must be supplied through the foods we eat.

Like carbohydrates, protein provides four calories per gram and can be burned as fuel. However, protein is used as an energy source only when carbohydrates aren't available. Protein is an expensive energy source because protein's first priorities are in building and repairing the body, not in fueling the body. This is why a balanced diet is so important. If adequate calories are eaten, and 20 percent of the calories are from protein, 50 to 60 percent from carbohydrates, and the rest from fat, protein will be saved for its most important jobs and not be wasted as a fuel source.

Some athletes want to believe that eating extra protein builds bigger muscles, but this is not the case. Once the protein requirement for muscle building is met, any extra protein is burned for fuel or stored as fat.

## Fat: Not a Diet Demon

For some time now fat has been maligned as a dietary evil, but in reality it is an important nutrient whose place in the diet is misunderstood. Fat in the body is necessary to absorb fat-soluble vitamins, protect internal organs, and keep us warm by providing insulation. Growing athletes should derive about 25 to 30 percent of their calories from fat.

---

## Cholesterol

Though it is sometimes confused with fat, cholesterol is *not* fat. Cholesterol is a fat-like substance that provides no calories, no energy, to the body. There are two kinds of cholesterol: dietary cholesterol and blood cholesterol. Dietary cholesterol is found only in foods of animal origin. When people are told they have "high cholesterol," they assume they need to limit their dietary cholesterol. But that is only part of the story. The focus is on the total diet—watching total fat intake, decreasing saturated fat, limiting cholesterol; you can't simplify it, which has confused people for years. It is a combination of total fat, saturated fat, dietary cholesterol, total calories, and of course, family history that affects your blood cholesterol.

---

Dietary fat is also important because it provides a feeling of satiety—it makes us feel full. Athletes who eat very low-fat diets have a hard time getting enough calories to support growth, and they always feel hungry. Of course, too much fat isn't good for anyone, and this is why fat gets a bad reputation. Fat is a very dense source of energy, providing nine calories per gram. Fat occurs naturally in food such as meat, whole-milk dairy products, nuts, and seeds. Many people get too much fat because of the fat added to food during its preparation. For instance, frying food in fat typically doubles its fat content and adds many empty calories. Snack foods such as chips, candy, and baked goods also pack many calories from fat.

Eating the right amount of fat doesn't make you fat. If an athlete is over-weight, fat should not be eliminated but modified. A fat-free diet for a grow-ing athlete typically has a negative effect on growth and performance.

## Vitamins and Minerals: The Body's Sparkplugs

Vitamins and minerals are the small but powerful nutrients found in many foods. They don't contain calories themselves but play a key role in process-ing calories from food. Their primary job is to protect the body from disease; build strong, healthy bones; and help the body use food properly.

Vitamins are either fat-soluble or water-soluble. Fat-soluble vitamins—A, D, E, and K—don't dissolve in water and can be stored in the body. If you take vitamin supplements, do not exceed 100 percent of the maximum amount recommended for these vitamins. Because they are fat-soluble, they can be stored in the liver and become toxic if taken in very large doses. Toxicity is not a problem if you get these vitamins through natural food sources. (See table 11.2 on page 117 for tips on choosing vitamin and mineral supplements.)

Water-soluble vitamins include vitamin C and the B vitamins: thiamin, riboflavin, niacin, $B_6$, $B_{12}$, and folic acid. These are called water-soluble because they dissolve in water. They cannot be stored in the body, and toxicity is rarely a problem. If you get too much, you generally eliminate them in urine.

# A Balancing Act

Between 50 and 60 percent of the calories in an athlete's diet should come from carbohydrates. Between 15 and 20 percent should come from protein. The remaining calories should come from fat. No one eats percentages, though, so understanding which foods contain carbohydrates, protein, and fat and how much of those foods to eat is the practical way to plan a healthy diet.

If you want to know the exact amount of nutrients required to be healthy, the Recommended Dietary Allowances (RDAs) have been established to state the amount of nutrients required to meet the needs of healthy people. The RDA will soon be replaced by the dietary reference intakes (DRI; see table 2.2). Neither of these standards has much practical significance when it comes to diet planning.

The food guide pyramid (figure 2.1) is the teaching tool designed by the United States government to provide Americans with an understanding of the basic foods that make up a healthy diet. It is a visual depiction of the types of food that should be included in the diet and the relative importance each type of food contributes to the total diet. The pyramid focuses on eating a balanced diet that includes a variety of foods.

**TABLE 2.2** Food and Nutrition Board, Institute of Medicine–
National Academy of Sciences Dietary Reference Intakes:
Recommended Intakes for Individuals, Vitamins and Elements

| Life stage group | Vitamin A (µg/d)[a] | Vitamin C (mg/d) | Vitamin D (µg/d)[b, c] | Vitamin E (mg/d)[d] | Vitamin K (µg/d) | Thiamin (mg/d) | Riboflavin (mg/d) |
|---|---|---|---|---|---|---|---|
| **Infants** | | | | | | | |
| 0-6 mo | 400* | 40* | 5* | 4* | 2.0* | 0.2* | 0.3* |
| 7-12 mo | 500* | 50* | 5* | 5* | 2.5* | 0.3* | 0.4* |
| **Children** | | | | | | | |
| 1-3 y | **300** | **15** | 5* | **6** | 30* | **0.5** | **0.5** |
| 4-8 y | **400** | **25** | 5* | **7** | 55* | **0.6** | **0.6** |
| **Males** | | | | | | | |
| 9-13 y | **600** | **45** | 5* | **11** | 60* | **0.9** | **0.9** |
| 14-18 y | **900** | **75** | 5* | **15** | 75* | **1.2** | **1.3** |
| 19-30 y | **900** | **90** | 5* | **15** | 120* | **1.2** | **1.3** |
| 31-50 y | **900** | **90** | 5* | **15** | 120* | **1.2** | **1.3** |
| 51-70 y | **900** | **90** | 10* | **15** | 120* | **1.2** | **1.3** |
| >70 y | **900** | **90** | 15* | **15** | 120* | **1.2** | **1.3** |
| **Females** | | | | | | | |
| 9-13 y | **600** | **45** | 5* | **11** | 60* | **0.9** | **0.9** |
| 14-18 y | **700** | **65** | 5* | **15** | 75* | **1.0** | **1.0** |
| 19-30 y | **700** | **75** | 5* | **15** | 90* | **1.1** | **1.1** |
| 31-50 y | **700** | **75** | 5* | **15** | 90* | **1.1** | **1.1** |
| 51-70 y | **700** | **75** | 10* | **15** | 90* | **1.1** | **1.1** |
| >70 y | **700** | **75** | 15* | **15** | 90* | **1.1** | **1.1** |
| **Pregnancy** | | | | | | | |
| ≤ 18 y | **750** | **80** | 5* | **15** | 75* | **1.4** | **1.4** |
| 19-30 y | **770** | **85** | 5* | **15** | 90* | **1.4** | **1.4** |
| 31-50 y | **770** | **85** | 5* | **15** | 90* | **1.4** | **1.4** |
| **Lactation** | | | | | | | |
| ≤ 18 y | **1,200** | **115** | 5* | **19** | 75* | **1.4** | **1.6** |
| 19-30 y | **1,300** | **120** | 5* | **19** | 90* | **1.4** | **1.6** |
| 31-50 y | **1,300** | **120** | 5* | **19** | 90* | **1.4** | **1.6** |

*Note:* This table (taken from the DRI reports—see www.nap.edu—presents Recommended Dietary Allowances (RDAs) in **bold type** and Adequate Intakes (AIs) in ordinary type followed by an asterisk (*). RDAs and AIs may both be used as goals for individual intake. RDAs are set to meet the needs of almost all (97-98 percent) individuals in a group. For healthy breastfed infants, the AI is the mean intake. The AI for other life stage and gender groups is believed to cover needs of all individuals in the group, but lack of data or uncertainty in the data prevent being able to specify with confidence the percentage of individuals covered by this intake.

*(Continued)*

TABLE 2.2 Continued

| Life stage group | Niacin (mg/d)[e] | Vitamin B$_6$ (mg/d) | Folate (µg/d)[f] | Vitamin B$_{12}$ (µg/d) | Pantothenic acid (mg/d) | Biotin (µg/d) | Choline (mg/d)[g] |
|---|---|---|---|---|---|---|---|
| **Infants** | | | | | | | |
| 0-6 mo | 2* | 0.1* | 65* | 0.4* | 1.7* | 5* | 125* |
| 7-12 mo | 4* | 0.3* | 80* | 0.5* | 1.8* | 6* | 150* |
| **Children** | | | | | | | |
| 1-3 y | 6 | 0.5 | 150 | 0.9 | 2* | 8* | 200* |
| 4-8 y | 8 | 0.6 | 200 | 1.2 | 3* | 12* | 250* |
| **Males** | | | | | | | |
| 9-13 y | 12 | 1.0 | 300 | 1.8 | 4* | 20* | 375* |
| 14-18 y | 16 | 1.3 | 400 | 2.4 | 5* | 25* | 550* |
| 19-30 y | 16 | 1.3 | 400 | 2.4 | 5* | 30* | 550* |
| 31-50 y | 16 | 1.3 | 400 | 2.4 | 5* | 30* | 550* |
| 51-70 y | 16 | 1.7 | 400 | 2.4[h] | 5* | 30* | 550* |
| >70 y | 16 | 1.7 | 400 | 2.4[h] | 5* | 30* | 550* |
| **Females** | | | | | | | |
| 9-13 y | 12 | 1.0 | 300 | 1.8 | 4* | 20* | 375* |
| 14-18 y | 14 | 1.2 | 400[i] | 2.4 | 5* | 25* | 400* |
| 19-30 y | 14 | 1.3 | 400[i] | 2.4 | 5* | 30* | 425* |
| 31-50 y | 14 | 1.3 | 400[i] | 2.4 | 5* | 30* | 425* |
| 51-70 y | 14 | 1.5 | 400 | 2.4[h] | 5* | 30* | 425* |
| >70 y | 14 | 1.5 | 400 | 2.4[h] | 5* | 30* | 425* |
| **Pregnancy** | | | | | | | |
| ≤ 18 y | 18 | 1.9 | 600[j] | 2.6 | 6* | 30* | 450* |
| 19-30 y | 18 | 1.9 | 600[j] | 2.6 | 6* | 30* | 450* |
| 31-50 y | 18 | 1.9 | 600[j] | 2.6 | 6* | 30* | 450* |
| **Lactation** | | | | | | | |
| ≤ 18 y | 17 | 2.0 | 500 | 2.8 | 7* | 35* | 550* |
| 19-30 y | 17 | 2.0 | 500 | 2.8 | 7* | 35* | 550* |
| 31-50 y | 17 | 2.0 | 500 | 2.8 | 7* | 35* | 550* |

[a]As retinol activity equivalents (RAEs). 1 RAE = 1 µg retinol, 12 µg β-carotene, 24 µg α-carotene, or 24 µg β-crypto-xanthin. To calculate RAEs from REs of provitamin A carotenoids in foods, divide the REs by 2. For preformed vitamin A in foods or supplements and for provitamin A carotenoids in supplements, 1 Re = 1 RAE.

[b]calciferol. 1 µg calciferol = 40 IU vitamin D.

[c]In the absence of adequate exposure to sunlight.

[d]As α-tocopherol. α-Tocopherol includes *RRR*-α-tocopherol, the only form of α-tocopherol that occurs naturally in foods, and the *2R*-stereoisomeric forms of α-tocopherol (*RRR*-, *RSR*-, *RRS*-, and *RSS*-α-tocopherol) that occur in fortified foods and supplements. It does not include the *2S*-stereoisomeric forms of α-tocopherol (*SRR*-, *SSR*-, *SRS*-, and *SSS*-α-tocopherol), also found in fortified foods and supplements.

[e]As niacin equivalents (NE). 1 mg of niacin = 60 mg of tryptophan; 0-6 months = preformed niacin (not NE).

| Life stage group | Calcium (mg/d) | Chromium (µg/d) | Copper (µg/d) | Fluoride (mg/d) | Iodine (µg/d) | Iron (mg/d) | Magnesium (mg/d) |
|---|---|---|---|---|---|---|---|
| **Infants** | | | | | | | |
| 0-6 mo | 210* | 0.2* | 200* | 0.01* | 110* | 0.27* | 30* |
| 7-12 mo | 270* | 5.5* | 220* | 0.5* | 130* | 11 | 75* |
| **Children** | | | | | | | |
| 1-3 y | 500* | 11* | 340 | 0.7* | 90 | 7 | 80 |
| 4-8 y | 800* | 15* | 440 | 1* | 90 | 10 | 130 |
| **Males** | | | | | | | |
| 9-13 y | 1,300* | 25* | 700 | 2* | 120 | 8 | 240 |
| 14-18 y | 1,300* | 35* | 890 | 3* | 150 | 11 | 410 |
| 19-30 y | 1,000* | 35* | 900 | 4* | 150 | 8 | 400 |
| 31-50 y | 1,000* | 35* | 900 | 4* | 150 | 8 | 420 |
| 51-70 y | 1,200* | 30* | 900 | 4* | 150 | 8 | 420 |
| >70 y | 1,200* | 30* | 900 | 4* | 150 | 8 | 420 |
| **Females** | | | | | | | |
| 9-13 y | 1,300* | 21* | 700 | 2* | 120 | 8 | 240 |
| 14-18 y | 1,300* | 24* | 890 | 3* | 150 | 15 | 360 |
| 19-30 y | 1,000* | 25* | 900 | 3* | 150 | 18 | 310 |
| 31-50 y | 1,000* | 25* | 900 | 3* | 150 | 18 | 320 |
| 51-70 y | 1,200* | 20* | 900 | 3* | 150 | 8 | 320 |
| >70 y | 1,200* | 20* | 900 | 3* | 150 | 8 | 320 |
| **Pregnancy** | | | | | | | |
| ≤ 18 y | 1,300* | 29* | 1,000 | 3* | 220 | 27 | 400 |
| 19-30 y | 1,000* | 30* | 1,000 | 3* | 220 | 27 | 350 |
| 31-50 y | 1,000* | 30* | 1,000 | 3* | 220 | 27 | 360 |
| **Lactation** | | | | | | | |
| ≤ 18 y | 1,300* | 44* | 1,300 | 3* | 290 | 10 | 360 |
| 19-30 y | 1,000* | 45* | 1,300 | 3* | 290 | 9 | 310 |
| 31-50 y | 1,000* | 45* | 1,300 | 3* | 290 | 9 | 320 |

fAs dietary folate equivalents (DFE). 1 DFE = 1 µg food folate = 0.6 µg of folic acid from fortified food or as a supplement consumed with food = 0.5 µg of a supplement taken on an empty stomach.

gAlthough AIs have been set for choline, there are few data to assess whether a dietary supply of choline is needed at all stages of the life cycle, and it may be that the choline requirement can be met by endogenous synthesis at some of these stages.

hBecause 10 to 30 percent of older people may malabsorb food-bound $B_{12}$, it is advisable for those older than 50 years to meet their RDA mainly by consuming foods fortified with $B_{12}$ or a supplement containing $B_{12}$.

iIn view of evidence linking folate intake with neural tube defects in the fetus, it is recommended that all women capable of becoming pregnant consume 400 µg from supplements or fortified foods in addition to intake of food folate from a varied diet.

*(Continued)*

**TABLE 2.2** Continued

| Life stage group | Manganese (mg/d) | Molybdenum (µg/d) | Phosphorus (mg/d) | Selenium (µg/d) | Zinc (mg/d) |
|---|---|---|---|---|---|
| **Infants** | | | | | |
| 0-6 mo | 0.003* | 2* | 100* | 15* | 2* |
| 7-12 mo | 0.6* | 3* | 275* | 20* | 3 |
| **Children** | | | | | |
| 1-3 y | 1.2* | 17 | 460 | 20 | 3 |
| 4-8 y | 1.5* | 22 | 500 | 30 | 5 |
| **Males** | | | | | |
| 9-13 y | 1.9* | 34 | 1,250 | 40 | 8 |
| 14-18 y | 2.2* | 43 | 1,250 | 55 | 11 |
| 19-30 y | 2.3* | 45 | 700 | 55 | 11 |
| 31-50 y | 2.3* | 45 | 700 | 55 | 11 |
| 51-70 y | 2.3* | 45 | 700 | 55 | 11 |
| >70 y | 2.3* | 45 | 700 | 55 | 11 |
| **Females** | | | | | |
| 9-13 y | 1.6* | 34 | 1,250 | 40 | 8 |
| 14-18 y | 1.6* | 43 | 1,250 | 55 | 9 |
| 19-30 y | 1.8* | 45 | 700 | 55 | 8 |
| 31-50 y | 1.8* | 45 | 700 | 55 | 8 |
| 51-70 y | 1.8* | 45 | 700 | 55 | 8 |
| >70 y | 1.8* | 45 | 700 | 55 | 8 |
| **Pregnancy** | | | | | |
| ≤ 18 y | 2.0* | 50 | 1,250 | 60 | 12 |
| 19-30 y | 2.0* | 50 | 700 | 60 | 11 |
| 31-50 y | 2.0* | 50 | 700 | 60 | 11 |
| **Lactation** | | | | | |
| ≤ 18 y | 2.6* | 50 | 1,250 | 70 | 13 |
| 19-30 y | 2.6* | 50 | 700 | 70 | 12 |
| 31-50 y | 2.6* | 50 | 700 | 70 | 12 |

It is assumed that women will continue consuming 400 mg from supplements or fortified food until their pregnancy is confirmed and they enter prenatal care, which ordinarily occurs after the end of the periconceptional period—the critical time for formation of the neural tube.

Reprinted, by permission, from *Dietary Reference Intakes*, 2002, (Washington, D.C.: National Academies Press).

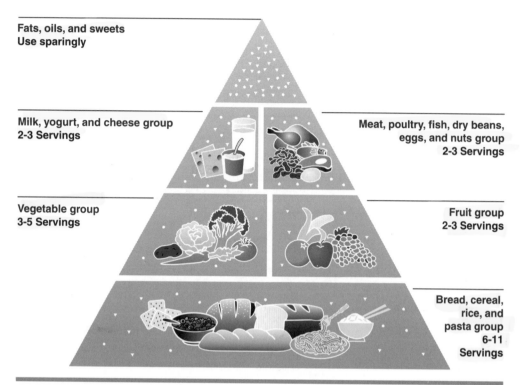

**Fats, oils, and sweets**
**Use sparingly**

**Milk, yogurt, and cheese group**
**2-3 Servings**

**Meat, poultry, fish, dry beans,**
**eggs, and nuts group**
**2-3 Servings**

**Vegetable group**
**3-5 Servings**

**Fruit group**
**2-3 Servings**

**Bread, cereal,**
**rice, and**
**pasta group**
**6-11**
**Servings**

***Figure 2.1*** Food guide pyramid.
Source: U.S. Department of Agriculture/U.S. Department of Health and Human Services.

The pyramid categorizes food into six groups depending on the nutrients the foods contain (figure 2.2). For instance, calcium-rich foods include milk, yogurt, and cheese. They are grouped together because they are rich in similar nutrients. The shape of the pyramid tells us that the foods at the base are needed in greater quantities than those at the top. Their place in the pyramid relative to other food shows the amount needed in the diet, not the importance of the food. All food groups are important, but some nutrients are needed in greater amounts.

The number of servings a person should eat from each group depends on activity level, age, and gender. The number of portions required by athletic children varies tremendously, but many find that they need more servings than are typically recommended.

One of the criticisms of the pyramid is that portion sizes are not realistic. Look closely at what is considered a serving size (table 2.3), then increase the number of servings as needed to meet the requirements of a growing athlete.

Grain foods form the base of the pyramid. These foods are rich in carbohydrates. The base of the pyramid emphasizes complex, not simple, carbohydrates. Simple carbohydrate foods—candy, cookies, soft drinks, and other

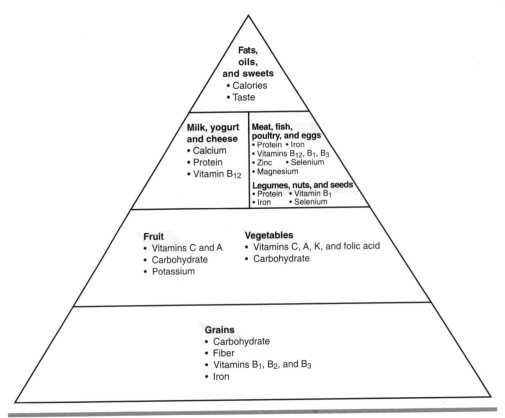

**Figure 2.2**   Nutrient pyramid.

sweets—contain only calories and few if any nutrients, so they are placed at the top of the pyramid.

Carbohydrates are the main source of fuel for the athlete, and most athletes have no problem meeting the recommended number of servings for grain foods. They should try to eat a good variety of foods, focusing on high-carbohydrate meals and snacks before and after exercise.

Fruits and vegetables are located right above the grains. These contain simple and complex carbohydrates and are packed with vitamins, minerals, and fluid. These foods are a gold mine for athletes. A serving of fruits or vegetables should be included with each meal and snack.

"Five a day" is considered the minimum number of servings of fruits and vegetables needed in a healthy diet. Looking at portion sizes, you'll see that five a day really isn't difficult to consume. Although fruit provides different nutrients than vegetables provide, choosing a variety of foods from either group works fine for children.

Fruit and veggies are portable, they rarely require refrigeration, and they taste great. Most fruit lends itself to pregame and recovery eating. Fruit can also be cut up and eaten during training and competition.

**TABLE 2.3    Portion Distortion**

| Pyramid portion | Real portions |
|---|---|
| Grain servings/calories | Real sizes/calories |
| ½ bagel/80<br>½ cup pasta/100<br>1 slice of bread/70 | ½ bagel/190<br>2 cups pasta/400<br>1 "hunk" of bread/200 |
| Fruit and vegetable servings/calories | |
| 1 apple/70<br>1 carrot/25 | Smoothie/400<br>Caesar salad/500 |
| Protein servings/calories | |
| Burger/180<br>Chicken breast/140 | Burger/400<br>Chicken breast/250 |
| Dairy servings/calories | |
| 1 cup of milk/80<br>1 oz of cheese/110 | About the same |
| Top of the pyramid servings/calories | |
| 2 tbsp salad dressing/100<br>½ cup of ice cream/150<br>2 cookies/100 | 1 ladle salad dressing/250<br>1 bowl of ice cream/400<br>½ sleeve of cookies/500 |

Adapted, by permission, from A. Litt, 2000, *The College Student's Guide to Eating Well on Campus*, (Bethesda, MD: Tulip Hill), 27.

Sitting on top of fruits and veggies in the pyramid are the protein and dairy foods. Protein is essential for muscle building and helps muscles recover after exercising. Along with protein, these food groups supply minerals such as iron, zinc, and calcium. To meet the suggested serving guidelines for dairy and protein, athletes should always include a serving of protein or a dairy-rich food in their meals. They should also eat a small amount of protein or dairy immediately after exercise. Serving sizes for protein are difficult to understand because they are given as ounces. See table 2.4 for an easy explanation of serving sizes.

At the top of the pyramid are the foods that offer calories with few nutrients. These foods are at the small tip of the pyramid for a good reason—we should eat far fewer of them than we eat of other foods. However, most diets can include these junk foods in an amount proportional to the rest of the diet.

Obviously, we eat junk food because it tastes good, not because it's good for us. It's unrealistic to think that young athletes will choose to avoid these foods completely. Those with very high calorie needs may be able to include more sweets in their diets.

The biggest drawback of using the pyramid as a teaching tool for athletes is that it ignores one of the most important nutrients: water. If athletes follow the fluid guidelines as outlined in chapter 3 and use information on appropriate portion sizes, the pyramid can be a solid foundation for planning a healthy and satisfying diet for growing athletes.

**TABLE 2.4** Serving Size Savvy

Just what does a three-ounce portion of meat look like? These examples might make it easier to visualize normal portions.

| Food group | Easy-to-understand portion or size |
|---|---|
| Grain group | |
| 1 cup of rice, pasta, or potatoes | Tennis ball |
| 1 pancake | Compact disc |
| 1 slice of bread | Cassette tape |
| ½ cup cooked rice | Cupcake wrapper full |
| 1 baked potato | Fist |
| Vegetable group | |
| ½ cup cooked vegetables | Scoop of ice cream |
| Fruit group | |
| ½ cup of fresh fruit | 7 cotton balls |
| ¼ cup raisins | Large egg |
| 1 medium-size fruit | Fist |
| Dairy group | |
| 1 oz cheese | Golf ball |
| 1 cup ice cream | Baseball |
| Protein group | |
| 2 tbsp peanut butter | Golf ball |
| 3 oz cooked meat or poultry | Deck of cards |
| 3 oz grilled or baked fish | Checkbook |
| Fats, oils, sweets, and snacks | |
| 1 tsp butter or margarine | Postage stamp |
| 2 tbsp salad dressing | Ping-pong ball |
| 1 oz chips or pretzels | 2 handfuls |

Adapted from Oregon State University Extension Family and Community Development.

# What to Do About Spirit Bags?

Teammates on girls' teams often bond by giving each other what they call "spirit bags," which appear in the girls' school lockers on game day. Included in the bags are treats such as candy bars, brownies, and chewy candies.

Although giving secret gifts to teammates is a nice idea, many girls don't want to eat the junk food in the bag and do so only because they don't want to appear ungrateful. A small amount of candy and junk is fine to eat, but spirit bags often go too far. A teenager concerned with diet and weight is faced with a dilemma: eat what's in the bag or give it away and possibly offend a teammate.

You might ask a team captain to set guidelines at the beginning of the season for how often bags can be given and what should be included in them. Suggest including sports drinks, bottled water, and *one* favorite candy bar or baked good. Or the bags could contain nonfood items such as socks, magazines, or hair accessories.

## Talking to Your Athlete About Nutrition Essentials

- Growing athletes have the same nutritional requirements as other children. They just need more of everything.

- Because their bodies are like fancy race cars, growing athletes need to take good care of their bodies, filling them with high-quality fuel.

- Carbohydrates, protein, and fat are the key calorie-producing nutrients. Vitamins, minerals, and water do not produce calories but are essential for proper body function.

- The food guide pyramid is an excellent tool for teaching athletes to include the correct amount of food in their diets. When using the pyramid, note portion sizes and keep in mind that the growing athlete often needs more servings than are recommended.

- An athlete's diet should be about 50 percent carbohydrate, 20 percent protein, and 30 percent fat. Following the food guide pyramid helps meet these percentages.

# Chapter 3

# FLUIDS FOR ATHLETES

Fluid is the most important nutrient for athletes. Some areas of sports nutrition may be open to debate, but hydration is not. Learning how much to drink, what to drink, and when to drink influences an athlete's performance more than any other dietary manipulation. Ignoring the proper guidelines impairs performance and might create dangerous, even life-threatening situations.

Drinking enough fluids requires developing and practicing a training plan. Like everything else in sports, proper practice makes perfect. As basic as drinking fluids may be, young athletes need to be taught that the water bottle may well be the most important part of their protective equipment. Well-hydrated athletes will feel better and play better.

## Importance of Fluids

The body needs fluids for digesting and absorbing food, transporting nutrients, removing metabolic wastes, and keeping joints lubricated. All of these functions are essential to a healthy body. For the athlete, fluids' most important and immediate function is regulating body temperature.

Fluid works as a coolant. When you exercise, your muscles produce extra heat. This is why you feel hot. To cool down and keep your body temperature in its natural range, you sweat. Sweat evaporates from your skin, allowing the body to cool down. Water lost through sweat needs to be continually replaced to keep the body running smoothly.

Temperature and humidity influence how much you sweat and the amount of fluid you need. When the weather is hot and dry, you may not realize the extent to which you sweat because it evaporates so quickly. When the weather is hot and humid, you sweat more, but less sweat evaporates. These conditions cause the body to heat up without an effective cooling mechanism. So although you're sweating, your body isn't getting much relief. At the opposite end of the spectrum, when you exercise at high altitudes, the dry air requires your body to "humidify" it. Because more water is needed for this, you must drink more, even when you're not feeling thirsty.

Environmental factors influence sweating for nearly everyone, but people sweat in different amounts. Some people sweat a lot, and others don't. Fit athletes tend to regulate their body temperature better by sweating more. Conditioned athletes thus need to replace fluids more often to compensate for higher sweat loss. Smaller bodies have less surface area and will sweat less than larger bodies.

Wearing breathable clothing encourages sweat to be "wicked" away, which allows you to sweat more. Wearing heavy equipment during a tough workout means your muscles may produce more heat and your skin may sweat more. The thing to remember is that the more you sweat, the more you need to drink.

## Dehydration: Debilitating and Deadly

When athletes don't drink enough, they may dehydrate, particularly in hot, humid conditions or during a hard workout. Dehydration results from inadequate fluid intake. It has a cumulative effect, so athletes should learn the early symptoms of dehydration to avoid the debilitating effects of severe dehydration. When severely dehydrated, the body compensates to protect itself from the lack of fluids by sweating less. This is when serious, even life-threatening, effects of dehydration occur (table 3.1).

When athletes are mildly dehydrated, their energy levels are diminished. They may feel sluggish or complain of a headache after practice. These early symptoms of dehydration are not serious, just bothersome. They are, however, insidious and occur before you begin to feel thirsty. Even mild dehydration adversely affects performance. As practice days pass without full and proper rehydration, the athlete and his or her performance are more and more affected.

It's natural for athletes to try to correct the problems of dehydration by grabbing a water bottle and drinking after practice. But this is like cramming

**TABLE 3.1　Dehydration Signs and Symptoms**

| Percentage dehydrated | Symptoms |
| --- | --- |
| 0-1% | Thirsty |
| 2-5% | Headache, fatigue, impaired performance, nausea, dry mouth, chills, clammy skin |
| 6% | Increased body temperature |
| 8% | Increased body temperature, dizziness, weakness |
| Over 8% | Heat stroke—sweating stops, high temperature, disorientation, death |

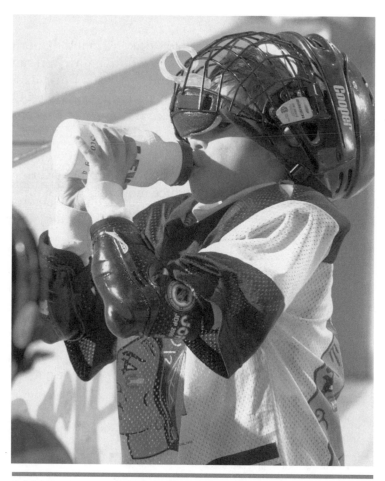

Athletes should drink water or sports drinks at regular intervals to stay hydrated during training and events. This is especially important for younger athletes, who are more susceptible to dehydration.

for a test. While some immediate relief is provided, drinking only after practice does not provide sufficient hydration. Proper hydration requires athletes to drink before, during, and after training. The fluid must be consumed—don't let your young athletes fool themselves into thinking they have cooled themselves off by pouring water over their heads. There's no problem with this superficial cooling method, but be sure they know that their bodies absorb needed fluid through the stomach, not the head!

A special word about working with younger athletes: Young children tend to sweat less and generate more heat. Their bodies are less efficient in transferring heat from their muscles to their skin. On top of that, children do not instinctively drink enough. Consequently, they are more susceptible to dehydration.

## How Much Is Enough?

How much does a growing athlete need to drink? To maintain normal body functions, the body needs about eight cups of fluid a day. You can get this amount from fluids you drink and from fluids naturally present in the food you eat. But fluid maintenance is only the beginning for athletes. Once they start moving, their bodies need much more fluid than the recommended eight cups. The amount they need is not naturally provided, so athletes need to follow guidelines to get enough.

To determine how much fluid they need, athletes should start with a practical assessment of evaluating their urine. They should urinate at least four times a day; their urine should be a pale yellow. If urine is concentrated and dark (the color of apple juice) or if they aren't urinating at least four times a day, they are dehydrated.

Another way of assessing fluid need is to teach athletes to monitor their fluid losses during exercise. Knowing the amount of fluid lost through activity helps them develop a method to replace lost fluids. To calculate fluid loss during exercise, follow the guidelines in table 3.2.

**TABLE 3.2     Determining Fluid Loss When Exercising**

| | |
|---|---|
| 1. Weigh yourself before exercising. | Weight _____ |
| 2. Weigh yourself after exercising. | Weight _____ |
| 3. Determine pounds lost. | _____ |
| 4. For each pound lost, drink at least three cups of fluid.* | |

*Actual fluid loss is two cups, but it isn't all absorbed.

Don't rely on thirst to tell you how much you need to drink. Once you feel thirsty, your hydration level has already been reduced. Athletes need to train themselves to drink well *before* they feel thirsty.

## Drinking By Plan

Many athletes are good at drinking at events but neglect their fluid needs when they are not competing. The American College of Sports Medicine (ACSM) has established guidelines for proper hydration. These guidelines, along with some practical tips, are shown in table 3.3. Athletes should follow this schedule for training and competing.

### Before Exercise

Athletes should drink at least 16 ounces of fluid, preferably water, about two hours before exercise. This amount is adequate for pre-event hydration. Drinking two hours ahead of exercise allows athletes ample time and opportunity to get rid of excess fluid through urination before exercise begins. It's

**TABLE 3.3     Fluid Goals for Athletes**

- Drink at least 16 ounces of water or other fluid 2 hours before an event.
- Top off by drinking 8 to 16 ounces of water 15 minutes before an event.
- Drink 5 to 10 ounces every 15 to 20 minutes of exercise. Use a sports beverage if exercise is longer than 60 minutes.
- Drink as much as possible within 15 minutes of the end of event or training.
- Continue to drink to replace fluids lost through sweat, plus more.

best to drink plain, cold water at this point. Cold beverages are absorbed better by the body. Water is the fluid of choice and the most important to consume throughout the day.

Beverages like sodas and fruit juices aren't recommended before training because of their high sugar content.These beverages might taste great, but they empty from the stomach slowly and don't provide enough hydration before or during events.

Every 15 minutes before the event, top off your fluid tank by sipping about four to eight ounces of cold drink. Starting off with a full tank lowers the risk of dehydration, and the fluids you have consumed move through the body more efficiently.

**During Exercise**

Whether they are exercising or competing, your goal is to keep your athletes' hydration levels high. The ACSM encourages drinking 5 to 10 ounces every 15 to 20 minutes during an event or training. Teach your athletes to drink at regular intervals, regardless of thirst. Many athletes don't like to drink during their events because they feel nauseated afterward. This often indicates that they are beginning to dehydrate and should be taken as a cue to drink more regularly.

Water is a perfect replacement fluid during exercise lasting less than 60 minutes. Water is also a reliable fluid choice to promote temperature regulation. However, when athletes exercise longer than an hour, or if they are involved in short but intense sessions, a sports beverage is a better choice than water.

Sports drinks contain carbohydrates, which are useful to working muscles that are running low on fuel. Other sweet fluids like soda and juice contain carbohydrates, but these higher concentrations of carbohydrates are not well absorbed or tolerated as a fluid source. Athletes may feel bloated, nauseated, or crampy after drinking these beverages. The lower carbohydrate concentration in a sports drink is better tolerated by the body.

Sports drinks also contain a small amount of sodium, which is useful because salt improves the taste and promotes drinking more. When athletes perspire, their sweat contains sodium, potassium, and chloride—electrolytes that must be replaced after exercise. But consuming the amounts found in sports drinks is not the best way to replenish the body with these nutrients. Athletes should regularly consume foods rich in potassium, such as bananas, tomato juice, and melons. For sodium and chloride replacement, they can use the salt shaker or eat and drink foods naturally high in sodium such as tomato juice, vegetable juice, and salted pretzels.

### After Exercise

Rehydration goals are to replace fluids as quickly as possible and get the muscles back in shape to perform. After exercise, athletes should be encouraged to drink as much as they can . . . and then more because absorption is quicker when fluid volume in the stomach is high. They should then try to drink to replace the fluids lost through sweating. It takes at least 16 ounces to replace each pound lost, but since the fluid isn't all absorbed, encourage your athletes to drink at least 24 ounces to allow for complete replacement and absorption of fluids lost.

## Beyond Water

High school athletes have access to many types of beverages, including soda, diet drinks, coffee, and alcohol. Though an occasional soda isn't bad, its high sugar concentration makes it a poor fluid replacement because it empties from the stomach too slowly to be useful. Diet drinks don't appear to have a negative effect on fluid replacement, but their general impact on children's health needs to be considered. There are conflicting reports regarding the safety of the artificial sweeteners in these drinks.

Of the sports drinks on the market, some are considered fluid replacements, and others are recovery fluids. Both contain carbohydrates. Recovery fluids also contain other nutrients, such as protein, and non-nutrients, such as caffeine and ergogenic aids considered helpful for recovering muscles.

Caffeine's value to an athlete's performance seems to depend on the individual. Some athletes feel jittery as a result of caffeine intake, whereas others say caffeine helps them stay focused. Most important to athletes is that caffeine is a diuretic, which promotes urination, so it is not a suitable choice for rehydration. Athletes should also know that the NCAA has established a legal caffeine limit of 15 micrograms/milliliter in urine tested. To determine how much caffeine this is, see table 3.4.

As for carbonated beverages, some athletes wonder whether the bubbles are easily tolerated by the body during exercise. Although tests show that carbonation doesn't seem to interfere with absorption rate, athletes may find that carbonated drinks make them feel full, thus limiting the amount they can drink.

Most teenagers these days can recite the dangers of underage drinking. What the teenage athlete needs to know, however, is how detrimental alcohol

**TABLE 3.4** Sources of Caffeine and Urine Levels Produced

| Product | Amount/dose | Equivalent in urine within 2 to 3 hours |
|---|---|---|
| 1 cup of coffee | 100 mg | 1.50 μg/ml |
| 1 coke or Diet Coke® | 45.6 mg | 0.68 μg/ml |
| 1 No-Doz® | 100 mg | 1.50 μg/ml |
| 1 Anacin® | 32 mg | 0.48 μg/ml |
| 1 Excedrin® | 65 mg | 0.97 μg/ml |

From: *Sports Medicine Advisor*, 2002, Caffeine and Athletic Performance.

can be to performance. Drinking interferes with every aspect of training and competing. From a fluid standpoint, alcohol does a poor job of regulating body temperature. Because of its effect on coordination, balance, and judgment, alcohol increases an athlete's risk of injury. Alcohol is always a poor choice for athletes.

# Keeping the Water Flowing and the Engine Running

Getting athletes to drink regularly may be as simple as providing them with a chart to monitor their intake (table 3.5). Have them track their intake to get a sense of what good hydration feels like. Encourage them to experiment with drinking bottles. Some players find a certain type of sports drink container makes it easier to drink more. See if they can tote one with them throughout the school day. If they prefer drinking a sports drink over drinking water, encourage them to drink both—the important thing is that they get plenty of fluids.

Some athletes find it easier to take just a mouthful of fluid at a time. If this is their style, let them know that an average mouthful is about one ounce. To meet sufficient intake levels, they need to take many mouthfuls. A problem with this style is that the smaller the volume of fluid in the stomach, the less efficient the body is at absorption. Drinking mouthfuls might do the job during exercise, but just before activity athletes should drink as much as they comfortably can so that their stomachs are full at the start and can efficiently deliver water as needed.

**TABLE 3.5    Hydration Diary**

| According to the latest research, here are the recommended drinking guidelines* to stay properly hydrated before, during and after exercise: | Before | During | After |
|---|---|---|---|
| | Drink **17-20 oz** approximately one hour before activity | Drink **7-10 oz** about every 15 minutes during activity | Drink at least **20 oz** of fluid per pound of weight loss within two hours** |

Determine the fluid you consume by "gulps" as one "gulp" usually equals about one ounce.

— 7 oz    Drink between 7-10 oz
— 10 oz   about every 15 minutes during activity

17 oz —

Drink 17-20 oz approximately one hour before activity

— 20 oz   Drink at least 20 oz of fluid per pound of weight loss within two hours after activity**

| Date | Activity | Duration/Weight | Reps/Sets | Fluid Intake (1 oz = 1 gulp) |
|---|---|---|---|---|
| | | | | |
| | | | | |
| | | | | |
| | | | | |

* Volume recommendations based on the National Athletic Trainers' Association (NATA) Position Statement: Fluid Replacement for Athletes, Casa, D. et al., J Athl. Train.

**To measure your fluid loss, weigh yourself before and after exercise. If you've lost a pound or more right after exercise, that's a fluid loss, and it means you need to hydrate.

# Talking to Your Athlete About Fluids

- Fluid is the most important nutrient for athletes.
- Proper hydration improves performance. Dehydration affects how athletes feel and impairs performance.
- Athletes should not use thirst as a cue to drink. If you are thirsty, you are already dehydrated.
- Learn to drink on schedule—before, during, and after physical activity.
- Water is the fluid of choice and the fluid to be consumed throughout the day.
- Sports drinks should be consumed during events lasting longer than 60 minutes.
- Sodas and fruit juice are okay in moderation but are not great choices because they have too much sugar for the body to use efficiently for fluid replacement.

# Chapter 4

# FUEL FOR MUSCLE DEVELOPMENT

Steak and eggs were once the breakfast of champions. Not so long ago, the training table was all about protein. Because strength is about bigger muscles, and muscles are made from protein, people believed eating a high-protein diet built bigger muscles. Now we know that muscle building isn't all about protein. Sufficient protein plus an appropriate complement of other foods plus a training program are what ultimately create muscles.

These days, athletes in nearly every sport are encouraged to cross-train. The soccer star lifts and runs; the field hockey player sprints and bench presses; the golfer runs to build up endurance. As athletes have learned to appreciate the value of cross-training, building muscle and increasing strength are now on everyone's list for improving athletic performance.

As we've learned more about feeding athletes and tweaking diets to take advantage of what each nutrient does best, protein indeed emerges as an important player. But it is just one player on a very large team.

## Protein: Of Prime Importance

Protein has several important functions in the body and is much more than just a muscle builder. Nails, hair, bones, and cells are all made from protein. Protein helps fight infection and regulates blood sugar and energy levels. Plus enzymes are made up of protein—which means protein is involved in every chemical reaction in the body.

As you learned in chapter 2, protein in food is made of small building blocks called amino acids. These acids are strung together in varying sequences to create the different proteins the body needs. Our bodies use 20 amino acids to make protein. Of those 20 acids, 9 are called *essential* because the body cannot make them, so we must get them from the food we eat. The other 11 acids are *nonessential* because they can be made in the body from other amino acids, carbohydrates, and nitrogen.

Foods contain different types of protein in varying amounts (table 4.1). Protein from animal sources including meat, fish, poultry, and dairy products is considered high-quality protein because it contains all the essential amino acids in a pattern that is useful to the body in creating new protein. Soy protein, though not an animal protein, is also considered a high-quality, or complete, protein.

Protein is found in plant-based food, too, but because one or more essential amino acids may be missing or limited in vegetables, these protein sources are of lower quality and called *incomplete*. A plant-based diet can still be nutritionally adequate, however (see information on vegetarian diets on page 37).

## Determining Protein Requirements

It's generally accepted that the Recommended Dietary Allowance (RDA)— the standard nutritionists use to assess adequacy of a diet—for protein is too low for athletes. Athletes need more protein than the general population (table 4.2). Still, it's possible for athletes to get enough protein by eating a balanced diet. Protein supplements may not be necessary, but they can be a convenient way to increase protein intake, especially for vegans (those who do not eat any animal flesh or animal byproducts).

It's fair to say a college football player has different nutritional needs from those of a high school football player; a long-distance runner will eat a diet different from that of a hockey player; a swimmer requires a protein intake different from what a diver needs. While these seem like obvious differences because of the sizes of the athletes and the sports they are playing, other factors also influence the amount of protein an athlete needs.

- **Condition of the athlete.** Early in a training program, the body is less efficient in converting protein to muscle. After the initial training phase, muscles get better at converting amino acids in the body into protein. Thus, the protein intake in the initial phase should be higher and then adjusted as necessary. Coaches and parents should pay attention to what their athletes eat during the preseason. Keeping protein levels high and attending to fluid and calorie intake help athletes feel better and perform better.

- **Total diet and timing.** Protein is a source of fuel, yielding four calories per gram (the same yield as carbohydrates), but being spent as calories is not protein's intended job. As mentioned earlier, protein is an expensive fuel source. If an athlete consumes adequate calories, protein can be saved for the important jobs unique to protein.

**TABLE 4.1** Food Sources of Protein

| Food | Serving | Protein (gm)/calories |
|------|---------|----------------------|
| Boneless, skinless chicken breast | ½ breast | 26/140 |
| Canned tuna | 3 oz (small can) | 22/100 |
| Skim milk | 8 oz | 8/80 |
| Vanilla yogurt | 6 oz (small carton) | 9/180 |
| Egg | 1 | 6/75 |
| Hard cheese | 1 oz (1-in. cube) | 7/110 |
| Cottage cheese | ½ cup | 14/80 |
| Sirloin steak | 6 oz | 51/308 |
| Hamburger | 4-oz patty | 33/292 |
| Flounder | 4 oz | 23/113 |
| Shrimp | 6 large | 8.5/45 |
| Cheese pizza | 1 slice | 14/200 |
| Nonmeat protein | | |
| Peanut butter | 2 tbsp | 8/188 |
| Chickpeas | 1/2 cup | 6/140 |
| Black beans | 1/2 cup | 7/162 |
| Pasta | 1-½ cup | 10/300 |
| Brown rice | 1 cup | 5/220 |
| White rice | 1 cup | 5/240 |
| Baked potato | 1 | 4/220 |
| Humus | 3 tbsp | 3/105 |
| Tofu | ½ cup | 20/183 |
| Veggie burger | 1 | 8/140 |
| Boca Burger® | 1 | 12/84 |
| Bagel | 1 large | 10/270 |
| Lentil soup | 1 mug | 9/140 |
| Minestrone soup | 1 mug | 5/120 |
| Black bean soup | 1 mug | 8/170 |
| Enriched soy beverage | 8 oz | 9/130 |
| Rice beverage | 8 oz | 1/90 |
| Tofu hot dog | 1 | 9/45 |
| Fast-food bean burrito | 1 | 13/370 |
| PowerBar® | 1 | 10/230 |
| Balance Bar® | 1 | 14/180 |
| Cliff Bar® | 1 | 12/250 |

Adapted, by permission, from A. Litt, 2000, *The College Student's Guide to Eating Well on Campus*, (Bethesda, MD: Tulip Hill), 125.

TABLE 4.2     Determining Your Protein Requirements
_____

**RDA for protein for average growing teenagers:**

|              | **Male** | **Female** |
|--------------|----------|------------|
| 11-14 yrs    | 45       | 46         |
| 15-18 yrs    | 59       | 44         |

**Protein requirements for athletes:**
Growing teenage athletes need about 0.8-0.9 grams of protein per pound of body weight. To determine the protein requirements of an athlete:

Multiply weight × 0.8 or 0.9 to determine grams of protein needed.

*Example:* 16-year-old Josh weighs 160 pounds.
160 × 0.8 = 128     160 × 0.9 = 144
Josh needs 128-144 grams of protein a day.

Protein requirements may be much higher for wrestlers, gymnasts, divers, and other athletes who eat a minimum number of calories. Because these athletes are often trying to maintain a low weight and eating a low-calorie diet, protein may be diverted from muscle building and repairing and used for energy instead.

Recovery foods—those foods eaten immediately after exercise—should include protein. Eating protein and carbohydrates within 15 minutes of completing a training or practice session allows muscles to rebuild and recover properly.

- **Sport played.** Athletes involved in strength and power sports look to increase their muscle size and strength. To build muscles, the body needs extra protein and a training program. Protein without proper training does not build muscles. Athletes should appreciate how training and diet complement each other. One without the other is bound to fail.

- **Athlete's age.** Protein needed by the growing athlete adds another layer to the protein requirement. Young athletes are building muscle, burning calories, *and* growing. They need to eat enough calories to first meet their growth needs.

Young athletes trying to bulk up often increase their protein intake because they think more protein means bigger muscles. Yes, protein is important for bulking up, but only when enough calories are ingested. High intakes of protein with inadequate calories means the protein will be diverted to other jobs, such as fueling the body.

Tony, a 10th grader preparing to try out for his high school lacrosse team, was interested in getting "ripped." He had started puberty at the age of 14 and was now 67 inches tall (75th percentile), 112 pounds (25th percentile), and growing on an average curve. Although he had played many sports, he had never been a superstar. He started going to a gym regularly, where he was instructed in proper techniques for strength and conditioning. He had also been told to eat as much protein as possible and had bought a protein-supplement powder. The powder was advertised as a "scientifically complete high-protein meal" and contained 280 calories, 2 grams of fat, 24 grams of carbohydrates, and 42 grams of protein. The instructions were to use it twice a day. Tony hadn't seen any difference and in fact was feeling hungrier than he had been before he started taking the supplement. At his initial assessment, he reported that he was using the powder to replace a healthy after-school snack—typically a tall glass of skim milk and either tuna fish or peanut butter on a large bagel.

## Original After-School Snack

|  | Calories | Protein | Fat | Carbohydrate |
|---|---|---|---|---|
| Bagel | 320 | 12 | 1 | 60 |
| Peanut butter | 188 | 8 | 16 | 6.5 |
| Skim milk | 160 | 17 | — | 24 |
| **Total** | **668** | **37** | **17** | **90.5** |
| With tuna/mayo instead of peanut butter | 273 | 30 | 17 | — |
| **Total** | **753** | **59** | **18** | **84** |

Tony also used the powder reluctantly in the evening, when he normally would have had a bowl of ice cream or cereal and milk. His old snacks tasted much better, and he preferred them to the supplement.

## Original Evening Snack

|  | Calories | Protein | Fat | Carbohydrate |
|---|---|---|---|---|
| Sugary cereal | 220 | 4 | 2 | 48 |
| Milk | 80 | 8 | — | 12 |
| **Total** | **300** | **12** | **2** | **60** |
| Ice cream | 360 | 5 | 24 | 33 |

After showing Tony this analysis, we decided that he needed to stick with his typical after-school snack, which was clearly a better source of calories and protein than the supplement he was taking. If he wanted to use the supplement in the evening, that was his choice, but it was not at all necessary given that his overall diet gave him more than enough protein for a young growing athlete. We also encouraged him to continue weight training and eating properly to promote muscle development now that his body was developmentally ready.

## Getting the Right Amount

Our diets are generally protein rich. Even the pickiest eater usually can get enough protein by eating ordinary food. But many athletes believe that a high-protein intake is so important that they purchase protein supplements, wrongly assuming that the more protein they eat, the bigger they will be. Many athletes also mistakenly believe that protein in supplements is superior to what they get from food. Protein supplements are not necessary in the diets of most high school athletes. And more is not better.

Some athletes also consider taking pure amino acid supplements, believing the body has a preference for using amino acids over the protein found in food. But there's no proof that amino acid supplements are useful, either.

Eating more protein than the body needs doesn't result in bigger, stronger muscles. Extra protein in the body is burned as fuel. What isn't burned is stored as fat. Overeating on protein doesn't build a lean body and, in fact, can ultimately lead to more stored fat.

If an athlete eats minimal calories, and most of them from protein, then the amount of carbohydrates his or her body gets is shortchanged. An athlete's body always depends on carbohydrates for fuel. Protein is not the first choice for fuel but is used if adequate carbohydrates aren't available.

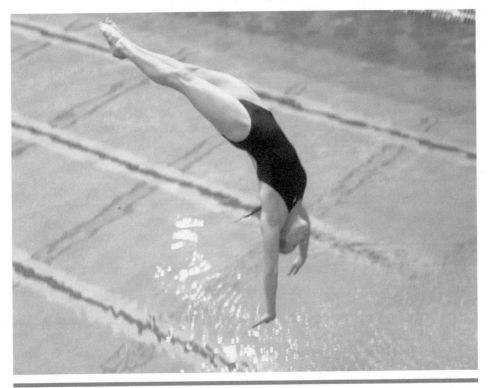

Protein often serves as an alternative fuel source for athletes who eat low-calorie diets, like wrestlers, gymnasts, and divers.

Protein and carbohydrates both contribute to glycogen stores. If an athlete is training or playing a sport longer than 60 minutes, glycogen stores deplete. When there is too much protein and not enough carbohydrates, the balance of nutrients preferred for maximizing glycogen stores isn't available, which affects power.

# Vegetarian Athletes

Vegetarianism is a popular choice for many young people. Children go vegetarian for many reasons. Some don't like the idea of eating anything that once had eyes, some follow an animal-free diet for religious reasons, and some believe vegetarianism is a healthier way to eat. For many kids, vegetarianism is a statement—a way to fit in or perhaps stand out.

Being vegetarian means different things to different people. Those who eliminate only red meat are generally called *semi-vegetarians*. Those who don't eat meat, fish, or fowl but do include dairy and eggs in their diet are called *lacto-ovo* vegetarians. There are variations within this type of vegetarianism as well, with some people being *lacto*, meaning they'll eat dairy but not eggs and some being *ovo*, meaning they'll eat eggs but not dairy. The most restrictive vegetarians are *vegans*, who won't eat anything of animal origin and often won't wear animal goods.

When an entire food group is eliminated from the diet, coaches or parents might express a legitimate concern that the diet doesn't meet the needs of the growing athlete. But with planning, a vegetarian diet is a healthy alternative. Simply eliminating meat does not necessarily pave the road to health, though.

The most important consideration when planning a healthy diet for vegetarians is to be sure the athlete eats enough calories. Once you're sure calorie needs are met, other nutrients to look at are protein, calcium, zinc, and iron. These nutrients are concentrated in animal foods, so eliminating animal foods means you need to find these nutrients in other sources.

The lacto-ovo vegetarian easily meets protein needs because dairy products and eggs are excellent sources of high-quality protein. As long as the lacto-ovo vegetarian eats the recommended number of servings, then protein intake should be fine (see figure 4.1).

The good news for vegans is that protein *can* be found in plant foods. However, protein from single plant sources are incomplete because one or more of the essential amino acids required by the body for protein building is limited or missing. Still, if plant proteins are properly combined, then the necessary amino acid pattern can be created. For instance, rice and beans both contain protein, but they each lack an essential amino acid. When eaten together, say in a bean burrito, they complement each other and make a complete protein.

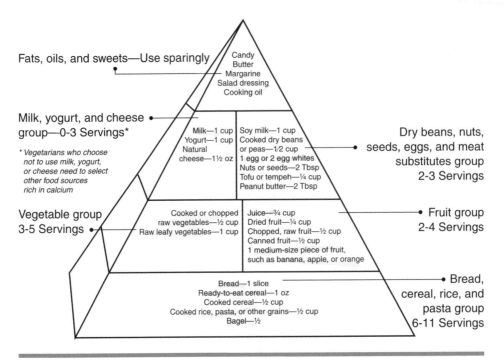

**Figure 4.1**  Vegetarian food pyramid.

Source: National Center for Nutrition and Dietetics: The American Dietetic Association; Based on the USDA Food Guide Pyramid. © ADAF 1997.

Nutritionists once stressed that complementary proteins must be eaten at the same time. We now know that as long as there are sufficient calories in the diet, complementary protein foods don't need to be eaten at the same time for the body to benefit from the amino acids they provide.

Calcium is an important nutrient for young female athletes. If dairy products are included in the diet, calcium needs should easily be met. Zinc and iron are concentrated in meat but are available in other foods (see table 4.3). Vegans also need to find a source of vitamin $B_{12}$. This vitamin is found naturally only in animal foods, so vegans must rely on foods that have $B_{12}$ added to them.

Some vegetarians eliminate meat only to realize later they don't know how to replace the lost calories. They fill up on junk food and end up with a poor diet. Many vegetarian athletes gain unwanted weight because they can't find the right mix of foods to satisfy them. Other vegetarians might use their diet to mask an underlying eating disorder. Following a vegetarian diet can give an eating-disordered teenager an excuse to eliminate entire food groups from the diet. In either situation, the diet that results is not a good one, neither for health nor performance. A coach or parent needs to observe changes in the athlete's eating habits and take the necessary steps to ensure a healthy diet.

**TABLE 4.3**  Food Sources of Calcium, Iron, and Zinc

| Food | Serving | Calcium (mg) |
| --- | --- | --- |
| Skim milk | 8 oz | 300 |
| Yogurt | 8-oz carton | 400 |
| Hard cheese | 1-in. cube | 200 |
| Cottage cheese | ½ cup | 75 |
| Cheese pizza | 1 slice | 150 |
| Broccoli | ½ cup cooked | 45 |
| Kale, collard greens | ½ cup cooked | 90 |
| Calcium-fortified orange juice | 8 oz | 300 |
| Calcium-fortified soy milk | 8 oz | 240 |
| Calcium-fortified string cheese | 1 piece | 250 |
| Calcium-fortified cereal | 1 cup | 250 |
| Ice cream, soft serve | 6 oz/small | 90-120 |
| Ice cream, hard | 1 scoop | 80-90 |
| Frozen yogurt, soft serve | 6 oz/small | 100-130 |

| Food | Serving | Iron (mg) | Zinc (mg) |
| --- | --- | --- | --- |
| Hamburger | 4-oz patty | 2.5 | 6 |
| Boneless chicken breast | 4 oz | .89 | .86 |
| Canned tuna | 3-oz can | 1.3 | .65 |
| Cereal | | | |
| Total® | 1 cup | 18 | .67 |
| Cheerios® | 1-¼ cup | 4.45 | .79 |
| Corn flakes | 1 cup | 1.8 | .9 |
| Bran flakes | ¾ cup | 18 | 3.75 |
| Cream of Wheat® | 1 cup, cooked | 9 | .31 |
| Instant oatmeal | 1 packet | 8.35 | .88 |
| Garbanzo beans | ½ cup | 1.65 | 1.25 |
| Lentil soup | 1 bowl | 4.2 | |
| Minestrone soup | 1 bowl | 1.4 | |

Devin, a 16-year-old football player, was turned off to eating meat after viewing a film in his environmental science class. At 6 feet, 2 inches and 170 pounds, he was always quite lean. He attended an all-boys' school, where his declaration to become a vegetarian raised the eyebrows of his football coach. His parents were meat eaters, and although they respected his decision, his choice concerned them. An initial assessment showed Devin's vegetarian diet to be inadequate in many nutrients, including protein and calcium. His initial intake and suggested modifications follow:

| Before | | After |
|---|---|---|
| **Breakfast** | | |
| Three Poptarts®/orange drink | | Four slices of toast with melted cheese |
| | | Calcium-fortified orange juice |
| School lunch | | |
| Two bagels with cream cheese | | Two bagels with peanut butter |
| Can of soda | | Two low-fat half-pint cartons of chocolate milk |
| Candy bar | | Yogurt |
| Ice cream bar | | Banana |
| Snack | | |
| Tortilla chips with salsa | | Two slices of pizza |
| Soda | | Water |
| Dinner | | |
| Pasta with butter | | Pasta with marinara sauce and grated cheese |
| Punch | | Skim milk |
| Garlic bread | | Garlic bread |
| | | Green salad |
| After dinner | | |
| Cookies | | Cookies and milk |
| **Totals** | | |
| Calories | 4,646 | 4,726 |
| Protein | 83 | 209 |
| Fat | 158 | 138 |
| Carbohydrates | 723 | 662 |
| Calcium | 969 | 3,158 |

Wanda, a 15-year-old competitive swimmer, had been a lacto-ovo vegetarian for about a year. She was always a picky eater and never drank milk or liked vegetables. She swam four mornings before school and three days after school and found that she was constantly hungry and gaining unwanted weight.

Plan I shows what she had been eating prior to receiving a nutrition consultation. Plan II shows the recommended diet she received at her consultation.

| Plan 1 | Plan 2 |
| --- | --- |
| **Before practice** | **Before practice** |
| Two cereal bars | Instant breakfast drink |
| | Cereal bar |
| **After practice** | **After practice** |
| Large bagel | Peanut butter and banana sandwich |
| Water | Sports drink |
| **Lunch** | **Lunch** |
| Baked potato stuffed with broccoli and melted cheese | Vegetarian sub with cheese, lettuce, and tomato |
| Bag of chips | Frozen yogurt |
| Soft-serve frozen yogurt | Water |
| **After school** | **After school** |
| Four large pretzels | Cereal and milk |
| Three handfuls of dry cereal | |
| Handful of gummy bears | |
| **Dinner** | **Dinner** |
| Pasta with marinara sauce | Bowl of minestrone |
| Mixed vegetables | Omelet |
| Italian bread | Two slices toast |
| | Wedge of watermelon |
| **After dinner** | |
| One cup of Teddy Grahams® | |
| Six sandwich-style cookies | |
| **Totals** | |
| 3,963 calories | 2,911 calories |
| 86 gm protein | 103 gm protein |
| 707 gm carbohydrate | 407 gm carbohydrate |
| 97 gm fat | 106 gm fat |

# Talking to Your Athlete About Protein

- Protein is needed for building and repairing muscles.
- Athletes need to eat more protein than nonathletes, but eating more protein than your body needs won't give you bigger muscles. Excess protein is used for energy or converted to fat.
- Protein needs can be met by eating a good diet. Protein supplements are not necessary for most young athletes.
- Meat, chicken, fish, eggs, soybeans, tofu, milk, yogurt, and cheese are excellent sources of high-quality protein.
- Beans, peas, lentils, nuts, seeds, and some grains also provide protein, but the quality is not the same. However, athletes can easily meet their protein needs on a meatless diet.
- Athletes who aren't in good shape and those just beginning an intense training program may need more protein earlier in the season.
- Eating a snack with protein and carbohydrates after a workout helps muscles recover faster.
- Athletes who eat a limited amount of calories, such as wrestlers, gymnasts, and some runners, may need more protein than other athletes need.
- Vegetarian diets can be planned to meet the needs of growing athletes.

# Chapter 5

# EATING FOR ENDURANCE TRAINING

Fuel for sport is all about carbohydrates. Carbohydrates are needed before, during, and after exercise. They supply immediate energy, are essential for maintaining fuel reserves, and help muscles recover from exercise. Cut them out of your diet, and you can cut yourself out of competition.

Carbohydrates are found in many forms in many foods. Knowing what foods and drinks provide carbohydrates and understanding how the body uses carbohydrates as fuel help you understand the best time to eat them. Endurance, performance, and recovery depend on the amount of carbohydrate-rich food you eat, the type of carbohydrates you eat, and when you eat them.

## Complex Story of Simple Carbohydrates

Carbohydrates are often classified as simple or complex. This tells us something about their structure, their nutrients, and their taste. All carbohydrates are made up of units of glucose, also called sugar. Simple carbohydrates are one or two units of glucose. They taste sweet, are easy to digest, and usually provide calories without other nutrients. Candy, soda, and most cookies are examples of simple carbohydrates.

Simple carbohydrates such as those found in candy, soda, and cookies are usually added to food in the form of sugar. Fruit is an example of a simple sugar found naturally in food. Fruit provides more than just calories. It is also a good source of vitamins and fiber.

Because they generally provide calories without other nutrients, simple carbohydrates are often called *empty calories* or the endearing term *junk food*. A diet of only simple carbohydrates is not a healthy diet because it doesn't contain necessary vitamins or minerals. That's not to say all simple carbohydrates are always bad. It's just that athletes need more nutrients than the average person, so eating only simple carbohydrates won't do. Strike a balance. It's naïve to think that young athletes are going to avoid junk food altogether. As noted earlier, there can be room for junk food within a healthy diet—but junk food should never be one's entire diet.

Complex carbohydrates have several units of glucose linked together. Complex carbohydrates (often called starch) are found in foods such as whole wheat bread, potatoes, pasta, and rice. In addition to calories, they provide vitamins, minerals, fiber, protein, and fat.

Regardless of the type of carbohydrate eaten, all are converted to glucose in the body and used as fuel. The body can store a limited amount of carbohydrate, called glycogen. This is a *fuel reserve*. When you eat more than your body can store or use, all carbohydrates are converted to fat and stored in the body.

## Gleaning Information From the Glycemic Index

In recent years, athletes have started paying attention to the glycemic index, or GI, which is another way carbohydrate foods are categorized. The GI is a ranking of foods from 0 to 100, determined in a laboratory measuring the blood glucose response from a particular food compared to a reference food. Foods are then categorized as high GI, moderate GI, or low GI (table 5.1).

Theoretically, a food's GI tells us something about the rate of digestion and absorption of its carbohydrates. High GI foods enter the bloodstream rapidly and are readily available as glucose, making them good choices during and after exercise. Low GI foods enter the blood more slowly, so they are better choices for pre-exercise, when you're looking for foods to sustain energy.

Is a laboratory test helpful to an athlete? The GI may be used as a guide, but only each individual athlete is in a position to determine which foods work best for his or her body. Regardless of what a laboratory might demonstrate, athletes should experiment with all carbohydrate foods to see which ones best meet their needs.

## Glycogen: The Staple for Stamina

When carbohydrates are eaten, they are broken down to glucose to be used immediately for energy. What isn't used for energy at that point is stored as glycogen. Glycogen can be stored in the muscles, and a lesser amount can be stored in the liver.

**TABLE 5.1    Glycemic Index**

*During or after exercise* (handwritten)    *Pre-exercise* (handwritten)

| High GI foods | Moderate GI foods | Low GI foods |
|---|---|---|
| Bagel | Pumpernickel bread | Pear |
| Grapefruit | Brown rice | Apple |
| Instant rice | Sweet potato | Pasta |
| Cereals | Corn | Milk |
|   Cheerios®, Crispix® | Peas | Yogurt |
|   Chex®, corn flakes, Grape Nuts® | Banana | Kidney beans |
|   Puffed cereals | Orange juice | Chickpeas |
|   Total® | Orange | Peanuts |
| Oatmeal | Apple juice | Sweet potato |
| Graham crackers | | |
| Crackers | | |
| Bread, white or whole wheat | | |
| Fruit | | |
| Raisins | | |
| Watermelon | | |
| Potato | | |
| Sports drink | | |
| Soda | | |
| Soda | | |

Adapted, by permission, from Powell, Holt and Brand-Miller, 2002, "International table of glycemic index and glycemic load values: 2002," *American Journal of Clinical Nutrition* 76(1): 5-56.

Glycogen stores determine how long an athlete can exercise without running out of gas. If glycogen stores are low, the duration and intensity of training are greatly reduced. Athletes participating in endurance sports such as distance running have long appreciated the value of glycogen. They know what it feels like to use up their stores and "hit the wall."

Glycogen stores are also valuable for athletes in sports such as football, soccer, and basketball, in which endurance is more in the form of intense, repeated bursts of energy. Fuel is used up quickly to support these activities, so glycogen stores become critical for maintaining energy throughout a game. To keep these stores loaded, athletes should "top off" by eating a carbohydrate-rich food before training and then refueling during breaks in play. This helps maintain a high energy level.

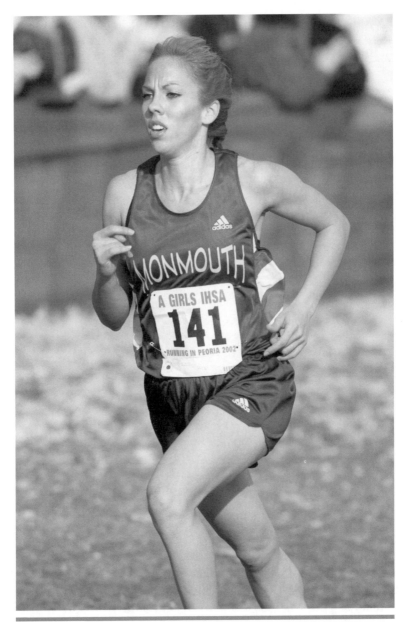

Carbohydrates stored as glycogen allow athletes like long-distance runners to exercise longer and harder.

## To Load or Not To Load?

The practice of training the muscles to store the maximum amount of glycogen for an event is known as carbohydrate loading. Research on athletes found that carbohydrate loading was effective in sustaining trained athletes for a longer duration when competing in endurance events.

Carbohydrate loading first became popular in the 1960s, mainly among distance athletes. It involved a complicated program starting one week before competition. Athletes depleted glycogen stores through intense exercise combined with a low carbohydrate intake. They then ate a high-carbohydrate diet while tapering their training.

The original method to reduce carbohydrate intake to prepare for the loading phase was abandoned because athletes felt so weak and drained without carbohydrates in their diets that they were unable to train. The need to deplete carbohydrate stores through intense exercise and carbohydrate restriction has been modified. Carbohydrate loading can be accomplished and appears to be just as effective when using a less extreme plan in which training is tapered and carbohydrate intake remains high.

Carbohydrate loading is effective when athletes are performing intense activity for 90 minutes or longer. It works only when athletes are already involved in endurance training. While loading might be helpful to the motivated high school distance runner regularly involved in endurance training, it is not necessary or effective for other types of athletes.

Encouraging young athletes to eat a high-carbohydrate pregame meal is valuable, but this is not carbohydrate loading. Young athletes believing they need to carbohydrate load before the next game should instead focus on eating a balanced pregame meal, drinking a carbohydrate beverage during the event, and eating a high-carbohydrate recovery snack.

Carbohydrate loading for a particular event is valuable only to very few young athletes, but eating a carbohydrate-rich diet regularly to increase glycogen stores is important for all athletes. Athletes can maximize glycogen storage by training and knowing what type of carbohydrates to eat and when to eat them.

The diet for training is as important, if not more important, than the diet for the actual event. Events generally last from 30 seconds (such as pole vault) to a few hours (such as a marathon), whereas training time is usually considerable for every sport. A short-distance swimmer swims miles in practice; a track and field athlete might spend hours training for a 10-second event; a rower is on the water for a long time every day practicing for an event that's very brief. The training diet for any of these athletes needs to be rich in carbohydrates to maximize glycogen stores during the intense training period that prepares the athlete for their event.

Even athletes participating in short-duration sports need to store glycogen to allow them to train well. The ability of athletes in any sport to maintain high levels of glycogen allows them to train harder, which usually influences performance.

## Carbohydrates: The Fatigue Buster

In season, athletes need to continually replace glycogen by eating a carbohydrate-rich diet. The more glycogen the muscles can store, the longer the athlete can exercise without feeling exhausted. If muscle glycogen is in a continuous state of being burned without being replaced, the athlete feels chronically tired and fatigued.

Carbohydrates are like medicine in the postworkout meal. Blood flow increases to exercised muscles, which allows muscle cells to "soak up" carbohydrates quickly and replace glycogen stores. For athletes involved in daily practices, a high-carbohydrate snack after training reloads muscle stores so that they can get out and do it again the next day. Without a doubt, eating carbohydrates after a tough workout is a real fatigue buster.

# Value of Fat

Athletes are accustomed to hearing about eating carbohydrates for fuel and eating protein for power—but what about fat? Endurance depends on eating a balanced diet. Fat is part of the package. Dietary fat and body fat each play a strategic role for the endurance athlete. However, many athletes often restrict their fat intake in an effort to reduce body fat. Limiting fat in the diet affects how carbohydrates are used for energy and ultimately affects energy level and performance.

Studies of endurance athletes suggest that some of the very low-fat diets consumed by some athletes actually impair performance. The amount of calories from fat is generally recommended to be 25 to 30 percent of the total calorie intake. This percentage range appears to be about right for athletes, too.

Helping athletes understand the importance of fat in their diets is a real challenge. Most athletes fear that eating fat will make them fat. The message they need is that eating a reasonable amount of fat will not increase body fat but will in fact help the body use its fuel sources effectively. It is better to include "good fats," such as those found naturally in avocados, olive oil, and nuts, rather than fat found in fried foods, whole-milk dairy products, heavily marbled meats, and processed baked goods and snack foods.

# Carbohydrate Phobia

High-protein, low-carbohydrate diets are currently in vogue for weight loss. But athletes needing to lose weight should *not* follow this type of diet. An athlete performing without carbohydrates is like a car running on kerosene—

you're in for a rough ride. Either training will be affected or performance will be affected. Without a regular and proper supply of carbohydrates, an athlete will be in a general state of fatigue.

Shelley is a 17-year-old field hockey player. She started the season a bit heavier than her normal weight and wanted to shed some pounds. She latched on to the diet trend of the day— high protein and no carbohydrates. She cut out all fruits and vegetables, traded her typical bagel and cream cheese breakfast for a protein bar, transformed lunch from two slices of pizza to a can of tuna, and had steak for dinner instead of pasta. She also eliminated from her diet most of the cookies, chips, candy, and pretzels she used to snack on throughout the day. She did start losing weight, but she was so tired all the time that her performance suffered.

A nutrition consultation showed Shelley that while her calorie intake wasn't bad, her intake of carbohydrates, the most important fuel for an athlete, was grossly inadequate. At first, Shelley was reluctant to add back carbohydrates because she was pleased with her weight. She then agreed to a compromise: She would return to consuming "safe" carbohydrates, such as fruits and vegetables, but would avoid the empty carbohydrates, such as chips and candy. She would replace her morning protein bar with cereal, fruit, and milk. She would have a tuna or chicken sandwich for lunch. Her dinner did not need to be a heaping plate of pasta, but she agreed to eat some potatoes or corn with her meat. Prior to her diet, she had been eating a great deal of empty carbohydrates. She was now encouraged to eat primarily vitamin-rich carbohydrates and far fewer sweets and chips. As a consequence of her compromise, her energy returned, her performance improved, and the unwanted extra weight stayed off.

If weight is an issue, look at the portion sizes of everything eaten (see table 2.3 on page 19). Eating too much of anything contributes to weight gain. Carbohydrates need to be part of a diet geared for high performance. Never cut out carbohydrates—instead, choose them wisely to support training and performance. Have sandwiches on bread rather than on large sub rolls or bagels; eat fruit rather than drinking juice; and cut way back on cookies and candy. Modify your carbohydrates, if needed, but never eliminate them.

High-carbohydrate meals such as pasta can remain a part of an athlete's diet, even when weight loss is a goal. Athletes concerned about gaining too much weight should follow guidelines for eating a reasonable portion of pasta and include it as part of a balanced diet, not the only meal in the diet.

# Talking to Your Athlete About Carbohydrates

- All athletes need a carbohydrate-rich diet. Carbohydrates provide immediate energy and can be stored as glycogen as a reserve fuel source.
- Simple carbohydrates taste sweet and are easily digested and absorbed. They provide calories without nutrients and are therefore known as junk foods or empty calories. Examples of simple carbohydrates are candy, cookies, sugar, and soda.
- Fruit is an example of a simple carbohydrate that does contain nutrients as well as calories.
- Complex carbohydrates are also referred to as starch. In addition to calories, they contain other nutrients. Examples of complex carbohydrates are whole wheat breads and cereals, pasta, potatoes, and rice.
- A healthy diet includes mainly complex carbohydrates, but including some simple carbohydrates is generally okay.
- A glycemic index tells us something about the rate at which carbohydrates are absorbed. Athletes may want to experiment with using the GI index to see whether it helps them sustain energy levels.
- Carbohydrate loading is effective only in events lasting at least 90 continuous minutes and only for athletes who are well trained to begin with.
- Eating carbohydrates within 15 minutes of exercising is essential for refueling glycogen stores. If glycogen stores are not replenished regularly, athletes will likely feel fatigued.
- Athletes need to include some fat in their diet to avoid fatigue.
- Low-carbohydrate diets designed for losing weight are inappropriate for athletes.

# Chapter 6

# TACTICS FOR GAINING WEIGHT

Weight gain can be a big deal for young athletes. It's not just about looking ripped—they want to be stronger, too. Yes, being buff is an ego boost, but for athletes playing sports such as football, basketball, lacrosse, hockey, and others, being bigger and stronger can be a huge advantage on the field.

For the many people struggling to lose weight, the idea of gaining weight sounds like a piece of cake. But for the young athlete on the go with little interest in food and no time to sit down and eat, gaining weight can be extremely frustrating. Fortunately, there are ways to help your athletes get in the best position to add some pounds if their bodies and minds are ready.

## Positive Gains

Gaining weight is a matter of creating a positive energy balance. This means eating more than you burn so that you have calories left over to create weight gain. Weight can be gained as muscle, fat, or a combination of the two. A growing body must eat enough to support growth and cover the calories it burns through exercise and daily tasks. Then the body needs to have some calories left over to build a bigger body. In some cases, we're talking about a lot of calories.

The amount of calories the body burns to function is known as the metabolic rate, which is very specific to each person. (For more on metabolic rate, see chapter 1.) Genes and body type affect metabolic rate and influence the body's propensity to gain weight.

The three genetic body types, or somatotypes, are shown in figure 6.1. Ectomorphs are generally long and lean with a small amount of muscle mass. They have a higher metabolism, burning more calories and making it a challenge to gain weight. The rounder, softer endomorph body type has

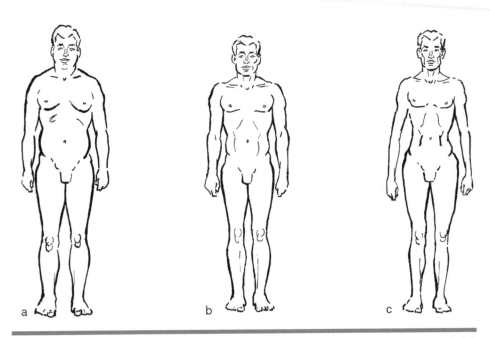

**Figure 6.1** Three genetic body types: *(a)* endomorph, *(b)* mesomorph, and *(c)* ectomorph.

a heavy bone structure and gains weight more easily. A mesomorph has a medium build, a large amount of muscle, and a medium to high metabolism. Most people are a blend of these body types, although some people are very clearly more one type than they are the others.

Both body type and metabolism play key roles in one's ease or difficulty in gaining weight. Some young athletes "run slow" and are prone to gaining weight simply because their metabolism sets them up for it. Other kids are just geared up a notch or two. They are fidgety and frenetic and always seem to be moving. This type of person has trouble gaining weight.

Active, growing children may need 3,000 calories or more a day just to maintain weight. To add a pound of muscle a week, they might need to add an extra 2,500 calories a week. Theoretically, if the child can eat an extra 500 calories every day, he or she will gain a pound in less than a week. But, the process is not as straightforward as it seems. When calories are added and exercise becomes more intense to increase muscle, the metabolic rate increases, thus requiring even more calories. And gaining muscle means increasing workouts in addition to eating more.

To consistently eat 3,500 calories or more a day is a struggle. For motivated athletes trying to gain weight, they will feel as if they are always eating—and they need to be in order to gain weight. The only ways to gain weight are to eat more, exercise regularly, and hope that genes and developmental readiness are on your side.

## Gaining Muscle

Athletes, particularly younger male athletes, don't just want to gain weight—they want to gain muscle. Protein is equated with muscle building and strength, so athletes looking to bulk up often focus on increasing the protein in their diets. However, as we discussed in chapter 4, weight gain is not only about adding protein to your diet.

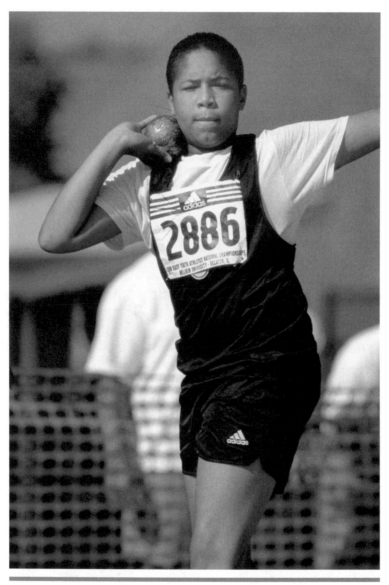

Many young male athletes want to gain muscle, but their bodies need to be developmentally ready before real muscle growth can occur.

Gaining muscle depends on the age of the athlete, genetic body type, proper strength training, and getting enough calories. Putting demands on the muscles through resistance training creates larger muscles, if there is ample protein and sufficient calories. Pile on developmental readiness, and you'll soon see a buffer body in the mirror. According to the American Academy of Pediatrics, "strength training programs for preadolescents and adolescents can be safe and effective if proper resistance training techniques and safety precautions are followed." Children beginning a program should be evaluated by a pediatrician beforehand and should also receive instructions from a professional familiar with the physical abilities and limitations of young children.

Puberty is as much responsible for muscle development as anything else. Without the right hormones available, real muscle definition won't be possible, and the buff look will be hard to come by. However, even before puberty it's appropriate and necessary to train young athletes to eat well and exercise right to get ready for when real muscle growth can occur.

## Gaining Weight and Performance

Does gaining weight really matter? Well, there's no question that in some sports, bigger and stronger are an advantage. But just gaining weight and being bigger don't ever guarantee improved performance. For weight gain to be useful, it needs to happen hand in hand with training. After all, a bigger kid won't necessarily be a faster kid.

Evidence exists that severe calorie restriction during puberty can limit growth. But will pushing calories create a taller person or create a more desired body type? Eating the best diet and working out offers an edge but will not change one's genes or developmental readiness. Trying to push weight gain in a body that is not developmentally ready simply will not work. What you can do is provide the child with support to eat a good diet and train correctly.

Jonathan, a 14-year-old competitive tennis player, was at the top of his game until he was bumped up to the under-16 age group. His speed and skill kept him competitive, but his size held him back. He wanted to eat better to get bigger and more powerful and thereby remain competitive. Like many competitive athletes, Jonathan focused on protein and supplements in his search for power. A nutrition consultation revealed that his calorie intake was marginal, mainly because he was using protein supplements that were not particularly caloric but were filling him up. He was advised to add calories first and to replace the protein powder drink he was drinking in the afternoon with a high-calorie smoothie.

# Balancing Weight-Gain Diets

It makes sense that to gain weight you should eat more. But eat more of what? French fries and doughnuts? Well, those foods might be included in moderation, but when you're gaining weight, you want to be sure the calories you get are from the right foods. Athletes need more calories than other people need, but they also should be sure that the calories they consume contain protein, fat, carbohydrates, and extra vitamins and minerals.

There are many commercial products on the market designed to promote weight gain, most of them advertised as "muscle builders." Some are totally worthless because all they contain is protein. For any weight gain supplement to be helpful, it must contain sufficient calories—and then it must *supplement* a diet rather than be a substitute for it. No research supports the idea that amino acids or protein delivered via a powder is at all useful in promoting muscle growth or weight gain unless there are sufficient calories in the powder as well.

Since dietary supplements are not regulated, some of the weight-gain products may contain potentially harmful or banned substances. Look carefully at the labels before purchasing weight-gain supplements. Learn which ingredients to avoid (chapter 11).

A young athlete can gain weight without using special products. If commercially prepared weight-gain supplements are used, they should contain extra calories and protein and should be taken within a good diet. But money might be better spent on a blender to make some tasty and much less expensive homemade smoothie recipes (see chapter 14).

# Boosting Calorie Intake

Gaining weight requires constant work. It means eating a lot and drinking a lot all of the time. Many underweight kids think they eat plenty, and maybe they do—but not with the consistency they need to gain weight. For some athletes to gain weight, they need to consider food as medicine and take it four to six times a day. They need to eat and drink when they aren't hungry.

A reasonable goal is for athletes to add an extra 300 to 400 calories a day to slowly promote a healthy weight gain. Young athletes may have an easier time adding calories if they eat five or six meals a day. Here are some strategies for adding additional calories.

*Increase portion sizes of what you're already eating.* Initially, this might mean eating until you feel uncomfortably full. Eventually, your stomach "stretches" and gets used to eating more, and a higher calorie intake is accomplished (table 6.1).

**TABLE 6.1     The Eat More Diet**

| Now | Cal | Eat more | Cal |
|---|---|---|---|
| 1 cup cereal with skim milk | 250 | Add banana to cereal | 350 |
| 4 oz orange juice | 60 | 8 oz orange juice | 120 |
| | | Slice toast with margarine and jelly | 185 |
| | | Hot cocoa | 110 |
| | | Granola bar | 130 |
| Turkey sandwich | 305 | Make sandwich on sub roll, add cheese | 750 |
| Apple | 100 | Apple | 100 |
| Water | | Add calorie-containing beverage | 140 |
| Chips | 150 | Chips | 150 |
| | | Yogurt or pudding | 100 |
| Cookies and milk | 450 | Cookies and milkshake | 665 |
| 2 beef tacos | 280 | 3 tacos with cheese | 495 |
| Handful tortilla chips | 140 | Handful tortilla chips | 140 |
| Water | | 10 oz juice or milk | 100 |
| Scoop ice cream | 265 | 2 scoops ice cream | 530 |
| | 2,000 | | 4,065 |

*Drinking calories is an effective way to increase calories.* Add a high-calorie beverage to each meal and snack. Use commercially prepared or homemade smoothies at least once a day in addition to eating five to six meals (table 6.2).

*Eat "denser" foods.* These are foods that contain more calories per mouthful, so you need to eat less to get more calories (see table 6.3). An example of a light food is your morning cereal, particularly "air-filled" cereals that might taste great and be good for you—but at 90 calories per cup, they take up valuable stomach space.

Fill a bag with 500 calories of trail mix, peanuts, or dried fruit at the beginning of the day and carry it around all day, eating small amounts here and there until the bag is empty.

*When preparing meals, add calorie-boosting extras* such as cheese to sandwiches, margarine or butter to vegetables, and potatoes and olive oil to rice and noodles. Throw in nuts, avocados, and dried fruit to salads and other dishes.

TABLE 6.2    Drinking More Calories

| Food | Serving | Calories |
|---|---|---|
| Soda | 12 oz | 140 |
| Orange juice | 8 oz | 110 |
| Cranberry juice | 8 oz | 120 |
| Grape juice | 8 oz | 155 |
| Apple juice | 8 oz | 120 |
| Commercial drinks (Snapple®, Fresh Samantha®) | 12 oz | 110-350 |
| Smoothies | 12 oz | 220-400 |
| Iced tea | 12 oz | 110-160 |
| Skim milk | 8 oz | 80 |
| 2% milk | 8 oz | 120 |
| Whole milk | 8 oz | 150 |
| Sports drink | 8 oz | 80 |
| Water | 8 oz | 0 |

TABLE 6.3    Dense Foods to Add to the Diet

| Eat this instead of . . . | Calories | . . . This | Calories |
|---|---|---|---|
| Cup of granola | 500 | Cup of Cheerios | 90 |
| Bag of peanuts | 170 | Bag of pretzels | 110 |
| Sandwich on a sub roll | 500 | Sandwich on bread | 300 |
| Bagel | 330 | English muffin | 130 |
| Blueberry muffin | 250 | Toast | 70 |
| Chocolate milk (1%) | 160 | Water | 0 |
| Trail mix | 220 | Cereal bar | 120 |

*Don't drink water before meals.* Although water is essential for athletes, they should not drink water before meals because this can give them a false sense of fullness.

## Talking to Your Athlete About Gaining Weight

- To gain weight, athletes need to eat consistently more than they are eating now.
- Athletes should eat three meals and three snacks and add a high-calorie beverage to all meals.
- Weight-gain supplements are often high in protein but not high enough in calories.
- Adding weight as muscle requires eating more of everything, training, and having a body that is developmentally ready to add muscle.
- Gaining in size does not guarantee that you'll be a better athlete in your sport.

# Chapter 7

# LESSONS ON LOSING WEIGHT

Many coaches and parents believe that losing weight can help athletes move better and become more competitive. This may or may not be true, but it *is* possible for growing athletes to make sensible changes in their diets that promote weight loss. However, dieting is not the way to do it.

Losing weight needs to be done right. When dieting is done wrong, the athlete feels the immediate effect of drained energy or stamina because of insufficient calories. Coaches and parents are often in a position to help young athletes make wise decisions as they strive to reach a weight that they're comfortable with. But adults walk a fine line when trying to help a young athlete slim down. There's gray area between what's healthy for the child and what's overly restrictive when it comes to eating choices. If not treated with care, the child could take any intervention from an adult as disapproval of their body type, which could deal a severe blow to self-esteem. Here are some ground rules when talking to children about their weight:

- Never discuss an athlete's weight or eating habits in public. If you're concerned about weight, talk about it with the athlete privately. If the subject is clearly uncomfortable for the athlete, don't push it. Revisit the discussion at another time.

- Do not publicly compare athletes' sizes, eating habits, or weight.

- Do not be the food police. It's a parent's job to offer a balanced diet and provide a healthy eating environment. (It is not a parent's job to diet for a child.)

- Don't weigh young athletes. Suggest that they keep track of their own weight, but don't require them to share the numbers.

## Is Weight Loss Appropriate?

As children develop through stages, they sometimes add weight in preparation for growth. Prepubescent girls must lay down extra fat for growth and menarche. They will typically look fleshier, even chubby. For boys, a "spare tire" around the middle often appears right before they hit a growth spurt. Weight loss during these critical stages in development is inappropriate and not recommended. Suggesting weight loss at this time could interfere with normal growth and be emotionally devastating.

Although it's tempting to want to "help" a child who appears to be gaining weight by suggesting a diet, restricting calories for a growing, athletic child is counterproductive. Children might interpret a suggestion that they eat less as deprivation, which could cause them to obsess about food and sneak-eat at every opportunity.

Why lose weight? Telling an invincible 12-year-old that he should lose weight to prevent premature heart disease when he is 40 falls on deaf ears. Health issues do not motivate children. However, children can appreciate the association of weight loss and moving quicker on the field.

Other than eyeballing a child's physique, how do you know if he or she needs to lose weight? Tools are available to determine healthy weight ranges. The number on the scale might be a starting point. Using that number, you can compare a young athlete's weight to the standard height and weight chart and get an idea of how the athlete's weight compares to the developed standards (figure 7.1).

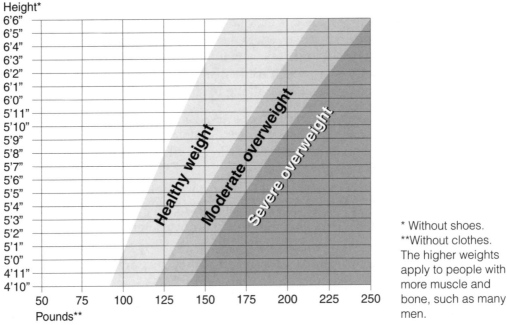

* Without shoes.
**Without clothes.
The higher weights apply to people with more muscle and bone, such as many men.

***Figure 7.1*** Standard height and weight chart.

Source: Report of the Dietary Guidelines Advisory Committee on the Dietary Guidelines for Americans, 1995, 23-24.

Body mass index (BMI) is another common standard used to determine a healthy weight range. BMI charts give a range that is associated with good health (figure 7.2).

To find an athlete's BMI, you'll need to know height and weight. Using both BMI and height–weight charts helps you determine whether a child's weight is too high when compared to accepted criteria. Use the Body Mass Index Calculator found at www.parents.com/tools/calc_bmi.jsp to figure out a child's BMI.

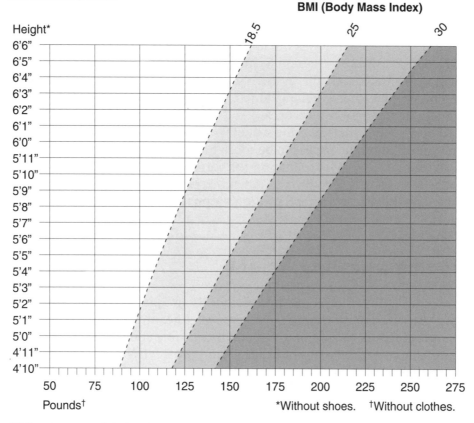

BMI measures weight in relation to height. The BMI ranges shown above are for adults. They are not exact ranges of healthy and unhealthy weights. However, they show that health risk increases at higher levels of overweight and obesity. Even within the healthy BMI range, weight gains can carry health risks for adults.

**Directions:** Find your weight on the bottom of the graph. Go straight up from that point until you come to the line that matches your height. Then look to find your weight group.

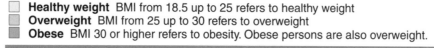

**Healthy weight** BMI from 18.5 up to 25 refers to healthy weight
**Overweight** BMI from 25 up to 30 refers to overweight
**Obese** BMI 30 or higher refers to obesity. Obese persons are also overweight.

*Figure 7.2* Body mass index chart.

Source: Report of the Dietary Guidelines Advisory Committee on the Dietary Guidelines for Americans, 2000, 3.

The flaw in both the height–weight tables and the BMI charts is that they don't take into account body fat. This is especially relevant for athletes who may actually weigh a considerable amount because they are muscular but have little excess body fat.

There are scientifically accurate methods to measure body fat using skinfold calipers, underwater weighing, and bioelectrical impedance (BIA). Skinfold calipers can be accurate and inexpensive but the procedure must be performed by someone skilled in the technique. BIA involves passing a small, harmless electrical signal through body tissue that assesses body fat versus muscle. New, less-expensive BIA machines are making their way out of research laboratories but are not yet widely available. Underwater weighing is the most accurate technique for measuring body fat, but this method is rarely available to the high school coach or concerned parent. One practical way of assessing body fat is simply to look for visible fat. Fat looks quite different from muscle.

Keep in mind that growing athletes should have some body fat. The amount of fat might appear to be more than is considered desirable if the young athlete's body is preparing for a growth spurt. Regardless of how tempted a coach or parent is to get rid of unsightly body fat on a young athlete, we never recommend putting prepubescent children on any sort of calorie-restricted diet.

## Finding a Healthy Weight

A good weight is about how an athlete feels and performs, not only about how he or she looks or what the scale says. A healthy weight means being able to eat without restricting, not being inflexible about food choices, and being able to eat a variety of healthy (and unhealthy) foods in a flexible, spontaneous way.

For girls who have started menstruating, a healthy weight should not interfere with a normal period. If a girl is restricting her calorie intake, her period might stop, which indicates that something could be wrong. Her weight could be too low, she might be overexercising, or she might not be eating properly.

Maintaining a realistic weight goal is confusing these days. People in our society are getting fatter, while the ideal body type promoted by the media is getting thinner. We've become accustomed to seeing ultrathin bodies in the movies, on television, and in magazines, and it's natural for us to measure ourselves against the images we see. When we don't measure up, we become unhappy with our own bodies. Yet the bodies we're admiring are often unhealthy. All of this makes it difficult to step back and figure out objectively what a good weight should be.

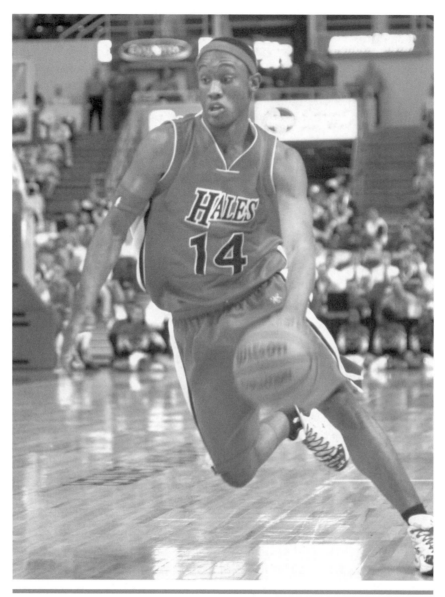

A healthy weight is one at which an athlete feels and performs his best.

Boys tend to be less critical of their bodies than girls are, but as athletes young boys are often seduced into weight-loss schemes with the hope of performing better or looking better. Boys can be quite sensitive about the layers of fat deposited before a growth spurt. Although some boys seem immune to the poking and joking about their weight, others are sensitive about it. Adults need to be just as careful with their comments about boys' bodies as they are about girls' bodies.

Bobby had always been big and was often told he'd make a good football player. The problem was that he was too big and had a hard time running. The summer before Bobby entered high school, he decided to improve his chances of making the football team. But he had two big dietary problems. For one thing, his parents were divorced. While one parent did a good job of planning meals for him, the other provided a lot of junk food and fast food. The other problem was that Bobby overheated so quickly that he had a hard time running.

Bobby met with a trainer who helped him gradually increase his running. A nutritionist helped his running by keeping him better hydrated via frequent water breaks.

To help Bobby's food intake, the nutritionist suggested the following guidelines to his parents.

## Meal Guidelines

- Drink a glass of water before eating any meal or snack.
- Eat all meals and snacks at a table, not while standing.
- Pace yourself. Eat slowly.
- Keep serving dishes off of the table.
- Abide by the 20-minute rule (described later in this chapter).
- Review fast-food menus before arriving and select meals ahead of time to avoid impulse selections.
- Order water at fast-food restaurants. Bring fruit to eat before your fast-food meal.
- Keep junk food less visible in the house.

# Weight-Loss Basics

Once you've determined that losing weight is an appropriate goal, let's look at how you can help your athlete safely and smartly reach that goal. Each year, Americans waste billions of dollars trying to lose weight. Get this straight: There is *no* miracle potion, pill, or gadget available to make weight loss easy. When infomercials try to tell you otherwise, turn them off. Losing weight and keeping it off are hard work, but it can be done.

Losing weight is about calories in (those eaten) and calories out (those needed for exercise, growing, and maintaining the body). There's no simple mathematical formula for losing weight, but computing the math is a place to start.

## How Much Do You Eat?

This is always tricky, because when people are asked to record their food intake, their record isn't an accurate reflection of their typical eating. But try it anyway. Commit to recording a typical food intake for three days. That means everything—the handful of dry cereal, the gulp of a smoothie, the crust from your friend's pizza. Use table 7.1 as your record keeper. Calorie books, food labels, and Internet diet programs are easily available to help you determine the number of calories in the food you record.

**TABLE 7.1    Keeping a Food Diary**

For an accurate picture of how much you're eating, you need to record everything you eat and drink. Write in your food diary on a typical school day and a typical weekend day to see your different eating patterns. While it might sound like a good idea to record for several days, most people get careless with their records after the first few days. Follow these steps to get the most reliable account:

1. Commit to recording on the days you decide. Don't try to plan "good" days.
2. Carry a small notebook with you. Record as soon as you have eaten. Waiting until you get home makes it easy to forget.
3. Record everything. This includes the spoonful of peanut butter you had while making your lunch for the next day, the five chips your friend shared with you, and the three caramels you had on the bus ride home from school.
4. Indicate whether you view this as a typical day or how it might be different if you weren't recording your intake.

**Example:**

| Time/place | Standing/sitting | Food eaten | Amount |
|------------|------------------|------------|--------|
| 7:00 | Bus to school | Cereal bar | Two |
| 10:12 | Standing | Soda | Three gulps |

## How Much Do You Burn?

Resting metabolic rate (RMR) is the number of calories that the body burns through involuntary body functions such as breathing, beating of the heart, lungs pumping, and so on. Your RMR is something like what a car engine does when the car is stopped at a stop sign. It idles, which burns some fuel, but it doesn't go anywhere. RMR is working 24-7 and accounts for 60 to 75 percent of calories burned daily. (For more on RMR, see chapter 1.) The remainder of metabolism is how many calories the body burns through exercising and moving about.

Age, body type, amount of muscle, and genetics influence metabolic rates. As a person reaches a mature age, metabolic rates slow down—obviously not a problem with growing athletes. More muscle means higher metabolism. And some people are simply born with a more revved-up fuel system. They burn more because their bodies idle at a higher gear.

An accepted formula for determining metabolic rate has been developed for adults, but it doesn't apply to growing children. Instead, a more arbitrary calorie guideline is used for children. (See table 1.1, page 2.)

To lose weight safely, children need to eat at least what they burn. They should never restrict their calories below the calorie guidelines. If they do, they may not get the nutrients they need and might be providing their bodies with too few calories.

## Creating a Safe Calorie Deficit

If you know how much a child eats and approximately how much he or she burns, you can create a calorie deficit that promotes weight loss. Although it might be tempting to dramatically cut back on calories to lose weight fast, doing so makes the athlete fatigued and interferes with performance. Instead, aim for a gradual weight loss accomplished by shaving calories that aren't necessary. See table 7.2 for suggestions on shaving calories.

**TABLE 7.2**    Shaving Calories

| Usual choice | Better choice | Calories saved |
|---|---|---|
| 8 oz 2% milk (120) | 8 oz skim milk (80) | 40 |
| 1 cup granola (460) | 1 cup Wheat Chex® (150) | 310 |
| Premium ice cream (280) | Breyers® ice cream (150) | 130 |
| Pizza Hut pepperoni pan pizza, 2 slices (700) | Cheese pizza, 2 slices (480) | 220 |
| Big Mac (560) | Cheeseburger (320) | 240 |
| Large fries (450) | Small fries (210) | 240 |
| 6-in. meatball sub (420) | 6-in. turkey sub (290) | 130 |
| KFC fried chicken breast (400) | Roast chicken breast (170) | 230 |

Adapted, by permission, from A. Litt, 2000, *The College Student's Guide to Eating Well on Campus*, (Bethesda, MD: Tulip Hill), 89.

# Evaluating Popular Diets

Putting a child on a diet is always a bad idea. The caloric needs of growing children vary tremendously. Diets are set at arbitrary calorie limits and fail to take into account a child's changing daily needs. Some days, they might need to eat more because they are active, whereas on other days they'll need fewer calories. Assigning a child a set number of calories to eat each day undermines his or her ability to self-regulate.

Diets are seductive and filled with hype—and they never work. When it comes to healthy eating, one size rarely fits all. To help an athlete lose weight and keep it off, an eating plan should be customized to match lifestyle, age, physical activity, and food preferences. Most eating plans are just plain common sense: Eat less, exercise more, and include all of the foods you need.

---

## Evaluating Diet Programs

When it comes to weight-loss programs, it's so easy to be seduced into believing everything you read. But before starting any diet, be sure to evaluate it objectively. If it sounds too good to be true, it is.

- Does the weight-loss plan require you to purchase special food? A healthy program should be based on foods available to you. Special products should not be required to make a program work. The plan should include kid-friendly food that can be eaten even at fast-food restaurants.

- Are your favorite foods included? You must be able to include those things you really love without feeling guilty about it. You might need to eat these foods in smaller portions or less often, but there should always be room for favorites.

- Does the plan take into account the caloric needs of growing athletes? Many commercial programs are too low in calories and set the stage for a restrictive eating program. The result may be weight loss, but it might be temporary because anything too restrictive will likely lead to bingeing. Too few calories affect a growing athlete's performance and could interfere with growth.

- Does the plan promise quick weight loss? As much as we would love to lose weight quickly, this is never a realistic goal. For some growing athletes, the goal may be weight maintenance; for others, the goal might be a slow weight loss (never to exceed two pounds a month for a growing child).

- Is the program affordable? Losing weight does not need to cost a lot of money. Special products should not be required.

---

Popular diet programs are too low in calories for teenagers and definitely too low in calories for young athletes. They are too restrictive and might promote muscle loss, which affects energy level and performance.

# Losing Weight Without Dieting

Restrictive diets don't work, but modifying eating does. Making subtle diet changes that won't feel like a diet is a helpful strategy. Teach your athletes to eat satisfying foods without overeating. Help them to include favorite foods, even if they aren't health promoting. Forbidden foods become more desirable.

Parents should not be food police. Refraining from comment can be especially difficult if a child is putting on weight, but parents should try. Of course parents are not discharged from helping their children reach a comfortable weight. But dieting for your children never works. Instead, help your children by employing the nondieting strategies that follow. They will benefit the entire family.

- **Don't drink calories.** High-calorie soft drinks, fruit juices, and smoothies should be eliminated from the diet of someone trying to lose extra weight. Even healthy beverages like fruit juice are very caloric (see table 6.2 on page 57). Drinking calories does not satisfy hunger. This means that a child can drink a 300-calorie soft drink (such as a super-size drink at a fast-food place) without it affecting his or her hunger level. Eating those same 300 calories is much more satisfying and healthy.

  As a rule, encourage young athletes to drink daily two to three servings of skim milk, one serving (six ounces) of fruit juice, and then water. Athletes have very high fluid needs, as we described in chapter 3. Water is the fluid of choice except during a game or event or immediately after a workout. A sports drink is often the best choice then.

- **Watch the extras.** Topping your salad with a ladle of dressing, adding pepperoni to pizza, or melting cheese on a baked potato quickly adds an extra 200 to 400 calories to a meal. It's fine to add spreads to toast, dressing to salad, and toppings to potatoes, but do so consciously.

- **Try the 20-minute rule.** If a growing athlete routinely wants a second helping, try enforcing the 20-minute rule. Ask the child to wait 20 minutes before getting a second helping. During this time, he or she can have his dessert if he wants. Usually, within 20 minutes the signal for being full has kicked in, and the extra helping of spaghetti isn't necessary, after all.

- **Add a snack to eliminate grazing.** Hungry children graze. They go from cupboard to refrigerator to freezer, never sitting and eating, yet often consuming more calories than if they sat down and ate an entire meal. Eliminate grazing by having satisfying snacks ready and visible. Soup, a sandwich, or cereal and milk may sound like more calories than a snack should be, but grazing calories always add up to more than that. Encourage your athlete to sit down and eat the snack. (See table 7.3.)

- **Face the food.** A lot of calories are eaten by the handful—in front of the television, walking through the supermarket, riding in a car. These calories add up quickly yet don't satisfy hunger. Always try to put food on a plate or in a bowl and use utensils to eat. Remember to "face the food."

- **Honor hunger and obey fullness.** It's always right to eat when you're hungry. Try to help young athletes think about eating when they're hungry and stopping when they're full. If a child asks for more food, don't say, "How could you possibly eat more?" Instead ask, "Are you still hungry?"

**TABLE 7.3**    Satisfying Snack Foods

For growing, active children snacks should be like mini-meals. Offering a really hungry child an apple as a snack just won't do it. Try one of these filling snacks to provide nutrients and discourage grazing.

- Bowl of cereal with fruit and milk
- Toasted English muffin with one tbsp peanut butter and one tbsp jelly, glass skim milk
- Half-cup cottage cheese and fruit
- Two toaster waffles with applesauce
- Two hard-boiled eggs with celery and carrots

- **Never skip a meal.** Children have an easier time when meals and snacks are scheduled. Eating should occur only at scheduled meal and snack times, with no grazing in between.

- **Slow down and enjoy the food.** Many children race through their eating. They race right past fullness to feeling stuffed. Children eating too fast will eat too much. If you can get your children to slow down their pace, they'll feel full sooner and will eat less.

- **Five a day . . . but don't eat anything you don't like.** Certain foods, especially fruits and vegetables, are high in nutrients and low in calories. Offer a fruit or vegetable at each meal. One thing: Don't go overboard in making children eat what they don't like. They end up feeling unsatisfied and will find something else to eat.

- **Include junk in a safe way.** Every diet, even with weight loss as a goal, needs to include foods that taste good but aren't necessarily good for us. To decrease the likelihood of overindulging in high-calorie, low-nutrient foods, try to include them with a meal at a time when hunger isn't overwhelming.

- **Create a thin eating environment.** To help your athlete at meal times, keep your serving dishes off the table. We're all tempted to eat more when food is right in front of us. Make eating a pure experience by turning off the TV and facing the food.

- **Cook thin.** Cooking thin does not mean compromising taste or flavor. There are ways to shave calories without shaving taste. Taste should never be compromised in a healthy diet. See table 7.4 for guidelines for cooking thin.

**TABLE 7.4    Cooking Thin Guidelines**

Limit recipes calling for fried foods. If a recipe calls for greasing a pan, "paint" it using olive oil on a pastry brush.

Bake, broil, grill, boil, microwave, or steam foods for best flavor without adding additional calories.

Before cooking, remove skin from poultry and trim visible fat from meat.

Invest in flavorful condiments such as mustard, vinegar, salsa, and horseradish.

Buttermilk and plain yogurt make great bases for marinades. They are low in calories and high in taste.

Learn to "poach" chicken and fish in foil to preserve moisture and taste without additional calories.

Invest in a steamer to steam vegetables and rice.

Purchase a good quality nonstick pan. Learn to "sauté" onions and garlic in the pan using little or no oil.

"Stretch" rich sauces by using a small amount on the side. Let children use the sauces for "dipping" rather than smothering a dish with the sauce.

Don't eliminate oil from a recipe. Just cut back gradually to determine how much is necessary to retain flavor.

# Talking to Your Athlete About Losing Weight

- Athletes should *never* diet. Most diets are too low in calories and set up a restrictive eating pattern that can't be maintained in a healthy way.
- A good weight is within a range—not one number on a scale or an amount a friend weighs.
- To lose weight, look critically at how much you eat and drink. Modify gradually.
- Many body types are acceptable—not just those the media promotes as ideal.
- A child who has not yet gone through puberty will store fat to make necessary developmental changes. Although the added weight might feel uncomfortable, it's a normal and necessary part of growth and development. Losing weight at this time is never recommended.

# Chapter 8

# DIETARY DETAILS FOR SPECIFIC SPORTS

The world of sports nutrition is often compartmentalized into endurance sports or power sports. Endurance sports such as running and soccer place a premium on carbohydrates, whereas power sports such as football and weightlifting are all about developing large, strong muscles. But no sport is only about power or only about endurance. Every athlete needs to be strong, and every athlete needs to fuel the body properly, whether it's to support intense training or a grueling tournament day.

When a sport is about stamina and endurance, athletes need to know the basics on fueling for a whole day of competition. Sports with short, all-out effort throughout a game require athletes to know how to replenish expended glycogen stores. For some sports, it is the training diet that's important, not what the athlete eats on game day. Depending on the training, the sport, and the events, an athlete needs to know what to eat and when to eat to get the most out of a well-rounded diet.

The short-term reward for young athletes is how they perform on game day, but adults recognize that the real prize is helping our youths maintain a great diet as well as optimal training and conditioning throughout the year. Ultimately, this allows our young athletes to develop sound training and eating habits to carry them through life.

Some nutrition goals are common to all sports. All young athletes need a balanced diet that meets calorie needs for growth, activity, and general health. Carbohydrates are always needed for fuel, protein for muscle building, and some fat to round out the calories and balance the diet. All athletes need enough vitamins and minerals to allow nutrients to be used properly. And of course all athletes need to be well hydrated. Despite some commonality across sports, each sport also presents unique circumstances in which athletes can benefit by following specific recommendations.

# Baseball and Softball

Baseball and softball are games with short bursts of activity and low-intensity activity that lasts several hours. For young athletes, the duration of the event might drain fuel reserves. Some athletes might lose their focus if they don't eat a small snack at some point during a long game.

Baseball and softball schedules often include several games a week, which leaves little time for muscles to recover. Players will easily fatigue if they don't drink enough and refuel properly during and after a game.

Because most baseball and softball games are played during the hot and humid seasons, it's especially important to instruct youngsters about drinking fluids. Catchers wear heavy gear and may have increased fluid requirements. Pitchers expend more energy in baseball and softball than other players do and must be coached to drink enough fluids to avoid dehydration.

## Training Diet

Gregory is a 13-year-old eighth grader playing select baseball. He practices two evenings a week and generally has three games a week. He is just starting to grow and is carrying around a little extra weight. His parents say he is a picky eater. Here is what we suggest for a typical school day with a 6:00 P.M. practice.

| **6:45 Breakfast** | **4:00 Snack** |
|---|---|
| Frosted flakes with skim milk and a banana | 2 slices of cheese pizza<br>Water |
| **10:45 Lunch** | **7:45 Dinner** |
| Peanut butter and jelly sandwich<br>Small bag of potato chips<br>Applesauce<br>Juice box | Hamburger on a bun<br>Corn on the cob<br>Baby carrots<br>Chocolate milk<br>Watermelon<br>Ice cream sandwich |

### Nutrition information

| | |
|---|---|
| Calories | 2,439 |
| Protein | 96 gm |
| Carbohydrates | 354 gm |
| Fat | 70 gm |

### Game Day

Depending on the time of the game, players should eat a regular meal either before or after the game.

- Encourage players to take advantage of the time between innings to drink water or a sports drink.
- Keep quick carbohydrate snacks (cut-up oranges, boxes of raisins, granola bars) available during innings.
- If the game is played away, bring snacks and drinks for the athletes.

# Basketball

Basketball players need it all: speed, strength, agility, and staying power. Fueling properly requires enough calories to sustain a long practice and long game, enough carbohydrates to fuel muscles, enough protein and fat to supply building blocks for muscle growth, and plenty of fluids.

Basketball games are fast paced, but there's time for players to hydrate and refuel. Players don't think about eating because they don't feel hungry when they're running up and down a court. Coaches can encourage refueling during halftime by having cut-up fruit or sports bars available for players to eat. Encouraging players to eat recovery foods after games and practice helps them stay in top form throughout the long season.

High school basketball players come in all shapes and sizes, so their calorie needs are quite different from those of younger players. Getting enough calories can be a challenge for some very tall, lean males, while a small, fast female might need to fuel carefully to get enough calories without bulking up.

### Training Diet

Sarah is a 10th grader playing varsity basketball. She is five feet, seven inches tall and maintains a healthy weight. She practices every day immediately after school unless she has a game and also plays or practices one weekend day. She has always been careful about her food choices and needs to make sure she eats enough.

| **7:00 Breakfast** | **3:00 Before practice** |
|---|---|
| 2 packages of instant oatmeal<br>Calcium-fortified orange juice | Banana, granola bar, water |
| | **5:00 After practice** |
| **12:00 Lunch** | Yogurt, graham crackers, water |
| Bagel with cheese, lettuce, and tomato<br>Apple<br>3 sandwich cookies<br>Water | **7:00 Dinner** |
| | Teriyaki chicken with rice and vegetables<br>Orange |
| | **9:00 Snack** |
| | Frozen yogurt |

**Nutrition information**

| | |
|---|---|
| Calories | 2,495 |
| Protein | 110 gm |
| Carbohydrates | 432 gm |
| Fat | 43 gm |

## Game Day

High school teams often play two to three games a week. Players need to work normal meals into their schedule to make sure they get their necessary nutrients.

- Eat a pregame meal at least three to four hours before tip-off to allow for digestion.
- One hour before tip-off, provide quick-energy carbohydrate foods such as sports drinks, sports bars, or fruit.
- Drink water or a sports drink during the game.
- Keep water bottles, sports drinks, sports bars, and cut-up fruit ready for halftime.
- At the end of games and practices, encourage players to cool down. Then recommend recovery foods such as peanut butter on crackers, apples and string cheese, or a sports drink and hard-boiled eggs.

# Football

Football is a game of short, intense activity played over several hours. Football players in most positions want to be big, so they tend to focus on protein intake to build muscle. While protein is important, adequate intake of carbohydrates is necessary for fueling muscles to meet the short bursts of explosive energy during football. These repetitive, intense efforts quickly drain glycogen. Teaching athletes to increase glycogen stores by eating carbohydrates and protein regularly and after workouts helps them maintain a high energy level throughout a game.

Football is unique in its variety of desired body types depending on the position played. Certain positions require very lean bodies to move fast and quick. Other positions favor big bodies. Regardless of the position, all players want to be muscular, and they all need to be fueled to run.

Sometimes large boys are encouraged to play football because of their size. Once on the playing field, they find they are in worse shape than they expected. Such athletes often need programs to help them get into playing condition. Although they strive to be bigger, increased weight alone isn't beneficial. They need increased muscle mass in order to improve their speed and agility.

Maintaining a high calorie intake during a long football season is difficult for some boys. Practice times are often scheduled after school, making it difficult to fit in the high-calorie snack they need. Coaches should encourage players to pack a small cooler with snack foods to eat before and after practice.

Football season starts during the dog days of summer. Coaches need to give their players very specific fluid guidelines to prevent dehydration. High sweat losses impair performance, fatigue players, and present serious conditions, particularly during two-a-day training in stifling weather.

## Training Diet

Roger is a ninth grader and a three-sport athlete. Along with playing football in the fall, he plays basketball in the winter and swims in the summer. He is growing rapidly and wants to bulk up for football. He has never been that interested in eating and often forgets to eat enough. To gain muscle and weight, he needs to eat more regularly.

| **Breakfast** | **Before practice** |
|---|---|
| 12 ounces orange juice<br>2 cups cereal with 2 cups of skim or 1 percent milk<br>2 slices of toast with butter or margarine and jelly | 1 banana<br>16 ounces of sports drink |
| **Midmorning snack** | **During two-hour practice** |
| 1 cup of granola in baggie<br>1 juice box | Water and 16 ounces of sports drink |
| **Lunch** | **After practice** |
| Deli meat sandwich on a large Kaiser roll (4 slices of turkey, ham, or roast beef)<br>16 ounces of juice or milk<br>1 piece of fruit<br>1 large chocolate chip cookie | 2 slices of string cheese, 2 mini bagels, juice box |
| | **Dinner** |
| | 3 cups of spaghetti, 3 meatballs<br>1 large slice of garlic bread<br>Salad with dressing<br>8 ounces of milk<br>Large scoop of ice cream |

**Nutrition information**

| Calories | 5,343 |
|---|---|
| Protein | 187 gm |
| Carbohydrates | 765 gm |
| Fat | 172 gm |

## Game Day

Football teams play in the evening and during the day. Often, a team meal is planned before a game, making game-day meal planning a bit easier.

- Eat a pregame meal at least three to four hours before kickoff. The pregame meal should be rich in carbohydrates and somewhat low in fat.
- Some players might want to eat a carbohydrate-rich snack within one hour of kickoff to fuel glycogen stores.
- Encourage players to drink during the game. They should drink a sports drink during the hot months.
- Players should have a postgame sports drink and a snack within 15 to 30 minutes.

# Hockey

Hockey is a fast-paced, high-intensity sport requiring all-out effort for repeated short intervals. Hockey is played in a cold, dry arena where players might dehydrate quickly without knowing it. Players wear heavy equipment that adds to the workload and fluid loss.

Hockey players are often looking to get bigger to stand up to the full contact of the sport. They must also be strong and fast. Hockey players have very high calorie needs. Some growing players have trouble keeping their weight on during the season.

Younger players often have less priority for ice time, so they sometimes have very early practices. They should eat something before practice and immediately after practice to get the calories required by this very demanding sport. Players not properly rested and fueled are at an increased risk for injury.

## Training Diet

Lance, a 12th grader, is hoping to play division I hockey. He would like to maintain his weight during hockey season, which he has had a hard time doing in previous seasons. He has four after-school practices and plays two games a week.

| **7:30 Breakfast** | **Dinner** |
|---|---|
| Bagel with cream cheese | 3 cups of pasta with meatballs |
| Orange juice | Caesar salad |
| | Italian bread |
| **11:45 Lunch** | Milk |
| 2 grilled chicken sandwiches | |
| French fries | **Snack** |
| Chocolate milkshake | 2 bowls of cereal |
| | Skim milk |
| **Snack** | Banana |
| Smoothie | |
| Energy bar | |

**Nutrition information**

| | |
|---|---|
| Calories | 4,754 |
| Protein | 204 gm |
| Carbohydrates | 641 gm |
| Fat | 160 gm |

### Game Day

Scheduling meals on game day can be a real challenge for hockey players; they frequently travel considerable distances to rinks, and often at odd times.

- Players should eat three to four hours before a game. Because games can be at unusual times, players might need to top off with a high-carbohydrate snack an hour before face-off.
- Every player should have a water bottle. Players sitting on the bench can also become dehydrated sitting in a cold, dry arena. Encourage fluid intake for all team members.
- Glycogen stores will be depleted after skating. Players need to eat within 15 to 30 minutes after a game.

# Soccer, Field Hockey, Lacrosse

These three sports are often played under similar conditions. Each game requires short, intense bursts of activity over a long game time. Players need

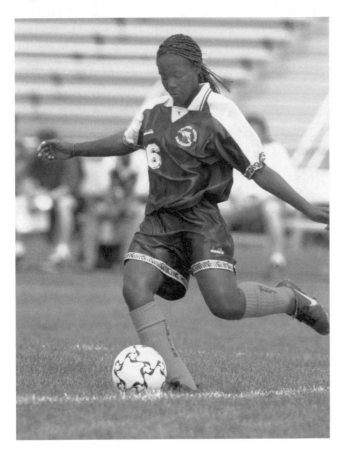

Soccer players require a carbohydrate-rich diet to keep players fueled for an entire game.

to be well fueled with a carbohydrate-rich diet in order to run as much as six miles a game. Games are divided into playing periods, so athletes have time to refuel. Keep sports drinks, water, and fruit available for players to eat during breaks.

Young athletes sometimes participate in weekend tournaments in which several games are played over a two- or three-day period. Give special attention to eating recovery foods so your athletes are in the best shape to participate the next day. Eating, drinking, and resting are essential to get them through their long schedules.

## Training Diets

Kate is a 17-year-old field hockey player. She practices four times a week from 5:00 to 6:30 P.M. Her weight is fine, but because she's up at 6:00 every morning to start school, she's very often feeling tired by the time practice rolls around. She needs to be sure she is well fueled for practice time.

| **Breakfast** | **Before practice** |
|---|---|
| Instant breakfast with milk | Sports drink and a box of raisins |
| English muffin with butter and jelly | **After practice** |
| **Lunch** | Energy bar and water |
| Tuna fish (water-packed) in pita bread | **Dinner** |
| Baby carrots | Barbecued chicken |
| Apple | Rice |
| Pretzels | Fruit salad |
| Water | Spinach |
| | Skim milk |

**Nutrition information**

| | |
|---|---|
| Calories | 2,330 |
| Protein | 117 gm |
| Carbohydrates | 351 gm |
| Fat | 52 gm |

Jim, an elite 11th-grade soccer player, is looking to get bigger and maintain his speed. When not practicing, he runs four miles a day and goes to the gym twice a week to lift weights. He's extremely lean and would like to bulk up.

| | |
|---|---|
| **7:30 Breakfast**<br>Cereal and milk<br><br>**12:00 Lunch**<br>2 peanut butter and jelly sandwiches<br>2 cartons of milk<br>2 large cookies<br><br>**3:30 Before practice**<br>2 bananas<br>2 sports drinks | **5:30 After practice**<br>Plain bagel<br>2 hard-boiled eggs<br>Water<br><br>**8:00 Dinner**<br>London broil<br>Mashed potatoes<br>Broccoli<br>2 dinner rolls with butter<br>Watermelon<br>Water<br><br>**10:00**<br>2 ice cream bars |

**Nutrition information**

| | |
|---|---|
| Calories | 4,862 |
| Protein | 226 gm |
| Carbohydrates | 657 gm |
| Fat | 163 gm |

## Game Day

Soccer players need to be well fueled but should allow sufficient time to digest meals. If they're playing in a weekend-long tournament, they should use their down time to stock up on carbohydrates.

- The pregame meal should be high in carbohydrates and consumed three to four hours before game time.
- Play is often continuous, but players should be coached to take advantage of rest to replace fluids and eat a source of carbohydrates.
- Refuel glycogen stores immediately postgame by eating a carbohydrate and protein snack.

# Rowing

Rowing, a sport gaining in popularity among high school athletes, involves long training sessions to increase endurance, improve technique, and build strength. The events are short, explosive exercises, but regattas are stretched out over weekends. Many rowers start land practice months before they hit the water. Overtraining can be a problem, especially if athletes are not properly fueled and rested.

A high-carbohydrate diet is needed for training. Practices are often at odd times. Early morning practice and late after-school practice interfere with meal times. Dehydration can be a problem during training. Boats need to remain as light as possible, so carrying extra fluids is often discouraged. Plus, rowers need both hands for rowing, which makes drinking awkward. Coaches should encourage frequent water breaks during training.

Before races, rowers might prefer to start with an empty stomach. The short explosive events may cause nausea if food has not digested. Allow three to four hours for the pre-event meal to digest.

Different body types are acceptable for crew. However, the coxswain is often striving for a specific weight. Lightweight boats are discouraged at the high school level. They can encourage rowers to "cut weight," which might lead to disordered eating behaviors.

Rowers work extremely hard. Many young male rowers have a difficult time getting in enough calories. Female rowers often have the opposite problem. They may gain weight initially in response to heavy training. They often need assistance with planning meals that have adequate calories to get them through training and keep them from overeating.

## Training Diet

Meg, a new rower, was finding that her increased activity was making her hungry all the time. She was gaining weight that she did not want or need to gain. She was famished after her afternoon practice and could not control her eating in the evening. Important diet changes for Meg included adding breakfast and an after-school snack.

| 6:30 Breakfast | 4:00 Snack |
|---|---|
| 2 slices of toast with peanut butter<br>Milk<br>Cut-up orange sections | Apple<br>2 pieces string cheese<br>Soup<br>Water |
| **11:15 Lunch** | **6:30 Dinner** |
| Turkey sandwich<br>Banana<br>Yogurt<br>Water | Chicken<br>Baked potato<br>Broccoli<br>Salad<br>Water |
| | **8:30 Snack** |
| | Cookies and milk |

**Nutrition information**

| | |
|---|---|
| Calories | 2,205 |
| Protein | 138 gm |
| Carbohydrates | 275 gm |
| Fat | 67 gm |

## Game Day

Race days are day-long events, with the actual event occurring hours after arriving at the race. Rowers need to plan carefully to keep their energy levels high.

- Eat the prerace meal at least three to four hours before the event.
- Choose a well-balanced meal.
- Drink fluids throughout the day.
- Eat or drink high-carbohydrate snacks throughout the day.

# Swimming

Swimmers spend a great deal of time training for events that often take less than a minute to complete. To get in the amount of training necessary, many swimmers are in the pool twice a day or practice in the pool and then have a session in the gym. For swimmers, nutrition goals are more important for optimal training diets rather than event-day diets.

Finding time to eat meals is a real challenge. Demanding training schedules interfere with meal times. Plus, most swimmers like to start their events with an empty stomach. Some swimmers need lots of time to digest foods to prevent cramping. Other swimmers do not encounter this problem and are able to eat and enter the pool without any problems. Swimmers often find that eating five or six small meals a day works better than the typical three meals a day.

Many competitive swimmers practice before school begins. It's difficult to eat at those predawn hours. Eating something small or drinking a sports beverage or fruit-based smoothie before practice will give them the energy they need for a productive session. After practice, they may go directly to school. Recovery foods after a morning practice will help them get through the day.

Swimmers have very high calorie needs. They often restrict their calories to gain the lean appearance they desire when wearing a swimming suit. Restricting calories is counterproductive and interferes with growth and energy level.

Because swimmers are in the water and may not feel themselves sweat, their fluid needs are often ignored. Swimmers should be encouraged to bring water bottles to practice and keep them at the end of lanes, drinking from them every chance they get.

## Training Diet

Jenny is a ninth grader who had been overweight in middle school. She swims three mornings a week and is always concerned about her weight. She needs to be well fueled to get through the day and strenuous practices, but she does not want to gain any weight.

| Preworkout snack | After school |
|---|---|
| 12 ounces of orange juice and banana | Yogurt<br>Apple<br>2 large pretzels |
| **After workout** | **Dinner** |
| Blueberry muffin<br>Skim milk | Grilled salmon<br>Baked sweet potato<br>1 cup of broccoli<br>1 roll with butter<br>Water<br>Oatmeal cookie<br>Skim milk |
| **Lunch at school** | |
| Peanut butter sandwich<br>Raisins<br>Granola bar<br>Water | |

**Nutrition information**

| | |
|---|---|
| Calories | 2,024 |
| Protein | 87 gm |
| Carbohydrates | 349 gm |
| Fat | 41 gm |

## Game Day

Game-day meals depend on when swimmers will warm up and when they swim in their event.

They should try to bring snacks to eat throughout the day, allowing ample time for swimming with an empty stomach.

- Swimmers prefer to start events with an empty stomach to prevent cramping.
- Choose one of the following meal patterns depending on time available to digest foods.

- Use sports bars, sports drinks, and gels between events to keep glycogen levels topped off without causing cramps.
- At meets, many swimmers rely on carbohydrate-containing beverages rather than solid food.

### Early Morning Meet (less than two hours to digest meals)

8 ounces orange juice
2 pieces of toast with jelly

### Mid-Day Meet (two to four hours to digest meals)

Grilled chicken sandwich
Banana
Sports drink

### Evening Meet (at least four hours to digest meals)

Regular mixed meal at least four hours before swim. Meal should include protein and carbohydrates and be low in fat.

# Track and Field and Cross Country

Track and field includes several events, most of which require short, explosive bursts of energy. Training, however, is intense and benefits from a high-carbohydrate diet to maintain glycogen stores.

Generally, the body type of athletes participating in track and field events is long and lean. Many of these athletes struggle to keep their weight down and often restrict their calorie intake. Fatigue from overtraining and undereating is common. The challenge for many of these athletes is to get enough calories to support long training sessions while keeping their bodies long and lean, as the sport seems to favor. Younger athletes in track and field might have a difficult time keeping their calorie intake high enough, whereas some of the older athletes don't eat enough.

## Training Diet

Emily, a high school junior, runs year-round. During track season, she sometimes "forgets" to eat and has been losing weight. She's tired all the time. Whether her forgetfulness is intentional to keep her weight down or a result of her focus on training is irrelevant. She needs a solid diet plan to stabilize her weight and boost her energy level.

| **6:45 Breakfast** | **5:30 After practice** |
|---|---|
| Cheerios | Protein bar |
| Skim milk | Orange |
| Strawberries | Water |
| **11:30 Lunch** | **7:00 Dinner** |
| Ham and cheese sandwich | Cheese ravioli |
| Pudding | Caesar salad |
| Banana | Skim milk |
| Water | **9:30 Snack** |
| **3:30 Before practice** | Ice cream |
| Sports drink | |

### Nutrition information

| | |
|---|---|
| Calories | 2,682 |
| Protein | 100 gm |
| Carbohydrates | 282 gm |
| Fat | 105 gm |

## Game Day

Athletes participating in several events at a meet should be sure to eat small, easy-to-digest meals throughout the day.

- Most athletes prefer to start with an empty stomach. The pre-event meal should be well digested before the event begins.
- Focus on recovery foods.

# Wrestling

Young wrestlers are among the most difficult to keep nourished. The wrestling community believes that wrestling at a lower body weight than is the normal weight for the athlete is advantageous. This puts young athletes in a desperate position to "make weight" for each match.

Wrestlers work to cut weight for a match by dehydrating themselves, purging, and drastically restricting their diets. Wrestlers hold to a common misconception that they can repair all the damage they've done to lose weight by eating well between weigh-in and competition. Unfortunately, this is not true. In fact, they could lose strength and their ability to concentrate through these methods to manipulate their weight.

Some state high school athletic associations are working to change the approach of cutting weight, but at this time it's still very much in vogue. Consequently, the adults in these athletes' lives will need to impress on them that they should make weight by wrestling at a weight that allows them to properly fuel their bodies (table 8.1).

Some wrestlers on restrictive diets become obsessed with food, which makes them likely candidates for eating disorders. As they grow older, their weight-cycling habits can also increase their risk for obesity. Because many of these athletes restrict their intakes, their diets could be lacking in several nutrients. Coaches and parents need to watch out for them and help them get enough nutrients to maintain health.

For wrestlers, the focus should be on their training diets, but more often it's on the calorie restrictions they employ leading up to a match. Because events are of short duration, the diet on the day of events is less important.

**TABLE 8.1**    Basal Caloric Requirements for High School Wrestlers

| Weight (lb.) | Basal calories |
| --- | --- |
| 98 | 1,544 |
| 107 | 1,674 |
| 115 | 1,728 |
| 123 | 1,781 |
| 130 | 1,824 |
| 137 | 1,910 |
| 145 | 1,952 |
| 155 | 2,017 |
| 165 | 2,081 |
| 175 | 2,100 |
| 185 | 2,206 |

To estimate additional calories needed for wrestling practice and daily school activities, multiply body weight by 11.3 kcal/hour/kg for wrestling practice and 1.5 kcal/hour/kg for school activities.

## Training Diet

Max, a 16-year-old wrestler, wanted to wrestle in the same class he had the previous year. The problem was that he had grown and gained some weight. Initially, he tried to restrict calorie intake to cut his weight, but he was constantly tired and thinking about food all the time. He was encouraged to wrestle at the next weight class up, at a weight of 145. This allowed him to eat more sensibly, and ultimately he was stronger and better prepared.

| **7:00 Breakfast** | **7:00 Dinner** |
|---|---|
| Scrambled egg white omelet | Flounder |
| English muffin with margarine | Broccoli |
| Orange | Baked potato |
| Skim milk | Dinner roll |
| | Skim milk |
| **12:00 Lunch** | |
| Grilled chicken sandwich | **10:00 Snack** |
| Skim milk | Applesauce |
| Apple | Ice pop |
| Yogurt | Yogurt |
| **4:00 Snack** | |
| Cereal and milk | |
| Banana | |

### Nutrition information

| Calories | 2,591 |
|---|---|
| Protein | 181 gm |
| Carbohydrates | 407 gm |
| Fat | 34 gm |

## Game Day

Encourage wrestlers to eat on game day, even if it means eating after a weigh-in. Entering any athletic event without fuel is not a smart game plan.

- Some wrestlers will not eat on the day they wrestle because of the timing of their mandatory weigh-in for their match. If possible, they should have a carbohydrate-rich, low-fat, low-protein meal before wrestling. They'll tolerate this better than a mixed meal.

- Some wrestlers find that drinking their calories works better for them than eating.

# Tennis

Tennis requires all systems to be working, sometimes for several hours under extreme conditions, such as 95-degree heat and high humidity. Tennis players strive to be lean, quick, strong, and agile. Maintaining a lighter body weight helps them move quickly across the court. In addition to long practices, they may spend much time weight training to build muscle and running to improve endurance.

Elite tennis players tend to be extremely fit, with very high calorie needs. They need adequate protein to build muscle, carbohydrates to fuel their glycogen stores, and enough fat to supply calories for endurance and fuel. Additionally, they must be very well hydrated because they're often playing for hours in the heat.

A key to fueling tennis players is keeping their glycogen stores full. They should bring food with them to matches so they can eat and drink as soon as a match is over. They may find sports bars a practical solution during their very long match days. These bars are easily digested and help keep energy levels topped off.

When they step onto a court for a match, tennis players never know if they're in for a quick 90 minutes or a long 5 hours. Consequently, tennis players should drink water all day long, on or off the court, to avoid dehydrating during a grueling match. Tell your players to prepare a large fluid bottle to bring on the court with them, gulping fluids at each changeover. They should drink sports drinks during their matches to maintain glucose levels.

In tennis, the training diet is as important as the game-day diet. While high school teams play in the fall or spring, elite tennis players are playing year-round. Depending on their level of competition, there may be very little off-season or other down time. Players competing and training regularly with only one or two days off a week should learn to eat and drink liberally on off days to compensate for their very full and calorie-demanding training.

## Training Diet

Liza is a 14-year-old elite tennis player. She plays or practices six days a week, traveling many weekends to tournaments out of town. She has an abbreviated school schedule to allow her to train. She is five feet three inches and extremely lean but has to work to maintain her energy level. A typical training day is shown on page 91.

| 7:30 Breakfast | 6:00 After practice |
|---|---|
| Egg white omelet<br>2 packages of instant oatmeal<br>Bagel<br>Chocolate milk | Power bar<br>Sports drink |
| **12:00 Lunch** | **7:30 Dinner** |
| Cheese pasta<br>Salad<br>Apple<br>Milk | Chicken, rice, vegetables<br>Baked potato<br>Salad<br>Water |
| **3:00 Before practice** | **8:30** |
| Orange<br>Lemonade<br>Bagel | Milk |

## Nutrition information

| Calories | 3,107 |
|---|---|
| Protein | 120 gm |
| Carbohydrates | 565 gm |
| Fat | 53 gm |

## Game Day

Matches are usually scheduled at more considerate times than in other sports. Still, tennis players should learn how much time they need to digest a full meal before going on the court.

- Try to eat a balanced meal within three hours of a match.
- Bring a fluid bottle on the court. Use a sports drink during matches lasting longer than an hour.
- Use days off to stock up on extra food.
- Refuel as soon as possible following a match.

# Gymnastics and Diving

Gymnastics and diving are sports in which skill and power are important. They are not characterized as endurance sports, and fuel reserves are not generally depleted, although training often takes place over several hours. Athletes in these sports need to take in enough calories to provide continuous fuel when training. Protein intake should be high enough to support their lean bodies, but calories need to be available for protein to be used properly. Like other athletes, gymnasts and divers need to be well hydrated, but many restrict fluids because they're concerned about their midriffs looking full.

The main nutrition challenge for divers and gymnasts is their emphasis on a particular body type. Typically, gymnasts and divers are very lean and muscular. Both males and females are concerned with body type, but because males mature later and natural body fat is lower, body concerns are more prevalent among females.

Many female athletes reach their peak in these sports early, sometimes before puberty. Early, intense training raises concern for properly nourishing a growing body. The very time that they need maximum calories for growth is when they are most concerned about their changing bodies and thus restrict their calorie intake. Calorie restriction interferes with strength and ability to stay focused, and in the long run it might interfere with their ultimate growth.

Because of the emphasis on a specific body type, gymnasts and divers are at high risk for developing eating disorders. Weigh-ins are discouraged. If coaches or parents notice a change in a young athlete's weight, they should address the matter immediately in private. Young divers and gymnasts need education and guidance to avoid the dieting mentality prevalent in their sports.

## Training Diet

Melissa, a 16-year-old diver, became concerned about her weight as the competitive season drew near. A small, muscular body type, she decided to lose weight. Although she lost a mere five pounds, this was 5 percent of her total weight. Unfortunately, she restricted her calories to lose that weight and consequently lost muscle, strength, and ability to remain focused. The following meal plan helped her follow a better plan during the season.

| 6:45 Breakfast | 3:00 Snack |
|---|---|
| 1 slice of toast with peanut butter<br>Skim milk latté<br>Applesauce | Apple<br>Teddy Grahams<br>Milk |
| **11:45 Lunch** | **6:00 Dinner** |
| Turkey pita sandwich<br>Pineapple chunks<br>Yogurt<br>Water | Chicken breast<br>Small baked sweet potato<br>Vegetable salad<br>Ice cream sandwich<br>Water |

**Nutrition information**

| | |
|---|---|
| Calories | 1,805 |
| Protein | 111 gm |
| Carbohydrates | 261 gm |
| Fat | 41 gm |

## Game Day

Gymnastics and diving meets often last hours, with events spaced out over the day. Athletes should know what they can eat throughout the day to provide fuel that is easily digested.

- Bring high-carbohydrate, easy-to-digest snacks, such as energy bars, cut-up fruit, and dried fruit.
- Learn how to sip liquids continuously to stay well hydrated without feeling "sloshy."
- Remind athletes that calorie restriction interferes with their ability to concentrate and affects their performance.

# Volleyball

Volleyball is a fast-paced game relying on speed, strength, and explosive power. Although volleyball might not be considered an endurance sport, maintaining glycogen stores is necessary for keeping players fueled for an entire match. As in all sports, hydration is important, especially if matches are being played outside.

Many different body types are found on volleyball teams. One concern among female players is the form-fitting shorts they wear. Females might feel self-conscious and attempt to restrict calories or resort to purging if they feel overweight or fat. Calorie needs are high, and restriction compromises energy level. Coach players to eat a balanced diet and take in enough fluids.

Training for volleyball can require practices two or three times a day. Players need to drink plenty of fluids and refuel as soon as they can after practice.

## Training Diet

Nora had never played volleyball before her freshman year in high school. She described herself as a "regular" athlete, loving sports but never the star on her team. As volleyball season started, she was surprised at how demanding the training was. She was not in very good shape to start and began running in addition to practicing with the team. Like many girls on the team, she watched what she ate. However, she was much more active now than she'd been before the season, and she soon realized she needed to eat enough food to maintain an energy level needed for her increased activity. She followed this plan during her intense training season.

| **6:00 Before morning run** | **2:30 Before practice** |
|---|---|
| 6 ounces of orange juice | Box of raisins |
| | Sports drink |
| **7:00 Breakfast** | |
| Scrambled eggs or 2 slices of cheese on an English muffin | **4:30 After practice** |
| Grapefruit juice | Bowl of cereal |
| Banana | Skim milk |
| | **7:00 Dinner** |
| **12:00 Lunch** | 2 to 3 slices pizza |
| Bagel and cream cheese | Green salad |
| Yogurt | Fruit cup |
| Raw vegetables | Ice cream cone |
| Brownie | |
| Water | |

### Nutrition information

| | |
|---|---|
| Calories | 2,718 |
| Protein | 109 gm |
| Carbohydrates | 417 gm |
| Fat | 78 gm |

## Game Day

Volleyball tournaments span over days, with many matches played throughout each day. Players should bring supplies to eat between matches. Determine the type and amount of food by the length of time they have between matches.

- Players may find it helpful to get up early enough to eat a high-energy breakfast, especially if they are traveling a distance to the tournament.
- Always pack plenty of food and beverages to last the day.
- Sports drinks will help maintain glucose levels.
- Eat and drink recovery foods, especially during multiday tournaments.

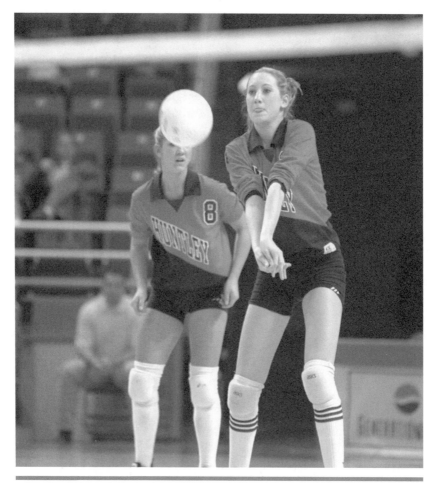

Volleyball players need to eat enough during tournaments to keep their energy levels up throughout the day.

## Talking to Your Athlete About Dietary Needs for Their Sport

- Nutrition goals common to all sports include the need to eat a balanced diet to meet caloric needs for growth, activity, and general health. Athletes always need carbohydrates for fuel, protein for muscle building, and fat to balance the calories.
- For many sports, the training diet is more important than the game-day diet. Eating well on game day does not make up for poor eating habits during the rest of the training period.
- Timing of meals is extremely individual. Some athletes find they need several hours to digest and absorb foods; others can eat or drink anything prior to game time.
- Do not experiment on game day.
- Pay attention to recovery foods.
- If athletes are involved in weekend-long events, be sure to plan. Pack a cooler with necessary food supplies.
- Athletes who have early morning practices should eat and drink before and after practice to keep their energy levels high throughout the school day.

# Chapter 9

# HIGH-PERFORMANCE MEAL PLANNING

Parents of athletes make tremendous sacrifices and concessions in their own lives to help their children succeed. Meal planning is no exception. The challenges of meal planning are knowing what kids should eat to give them the most energy, knowing when they can eat meals and snacks so that the food is used in a beneficial way, and managing the time and logistics to actually eat what is planned.

Feeding athletes might mean serving food at odd times to accommodate a demanding training schedule. It might mean sharing lunch together in the car on the way to a game so there's enough time for proper digestion. And it might mean setting your own alarm clock 30 minutes early to sit with your athletes as they eat a much-needed breakfast to get them through the day.

As a parent (or guardian), you're in charge of the meals you serve at home. You're also responsible for teaching your young athlete to make smart choices away from home. The benefit of following meal guidelines is that everyone eats better—not just your athlete but the entire family.

## Three Meals and Counting

Many schools start way too early for the natural clocks of children. Children often drag themselves out of bed with little time or desire to eat breakfast. When hunger hits, say about third period, they're stuck in class. Then there is the blur of lunch. Since many busy athletes have little free time to socialize, lunch is more often about friends than about food (which, by the way, is high-fat fare in many school cafeterias).

As classes drag on through the afternoon and they can barely keep their eyes open, young athletes have a grueling practice ahead of them, with little time to digest any real fuel. This leaves them with a rushed family dinner (if they're lucky), followed by homework, a shower, and maybe a little time to phone or e-mail friends before bed.

## Break the Fast

Your first job is to help your growing athlete (and other children) start the day strong. Breakfast doesn't have to be big, and it doesn't have to be breakfast food. Breakfast just needs to break the fast, preferably within an hour of rising. In a perfect world, families would wake up together and sit down to a healthy, calm, enjoyable breakfast. In our real world, alarm clocks go off at different times, parents are putting themselves together for work, and kids are flying out the door to catch an early bus. If you're going to raise breakfast-eating children, you might need to get up early and eat breakfast with them.

Breakfast can be a real struggle but is extremely important for the athlete getting up for early morning practice before going directly to school. Liquid breakfasts, such as a homemade or commercially purchased smoothie (see chapter 14 for recipes); a breakfast bar and juice; or just a piece of fruit on the way to practice might be all they feel like eating this early in the day. Whatever they can get down is better than not eating at all.

Athletes need to eat as soon as they can after a morning practice to refuel their muscles. With muscles fed, they will feel better physically and have more energy for the rest of the day. Postworkout breakfasts will most likely be eaten in the car. Think out of the box. Anything works, be it a traditional breakfast food or not. (See table 9.1 for breakfast suggestions.)

## Brown Bag Lunch

During the school year, lunch is the one meal that doesn't interfere with practice. Encourage your young athlete to take advantage of the opportunity and eat well while they have the time. Many athletes are busy most of the day, so lunch might be a time to relax, socialize, and just hang out. School cafeterias vary tremendously in what foods are offered and how healthy they are. As a coach, you can be very influential if you review the menu with your team and make recommendations. Good lunch choices (available in most school cafeterias) include sandwiches, soups, salads, fruit, and dessert. Encourage young athletes to bring their lunch to school, if this is an option. Packed lunches tend to be more economical, more healthy, and more efficient (because time isn't wasted standing in line).

Parents should help their child organize lunch the night before (table 9.2). By eighth grade, the lunch box has been replaced by a brown paper bag, so reusable ice packs don't usually make it back home. Freeze a water bottle or box drink the night before—this keeps the entire lunch cool and makes sure your child has something to drink.

**TABLE 9.1    Breakfast in a Bag**

A balance of protein, carbohydrates, and fat is necessary for starting the day strong. Add skim milk or hot chocolate made with skim milk or 100 percent fruit juice to any of these breakfast ideas. If carrying breakfast, freeze a box drink the night before, buy milk in box drinks, or pour hot or cold beverages into a thermos.

| |
|---|
| Peanut butter on an English muffin |
| Frozen waffles and applesauce |
| Cold cereal and fruit |
| Instant hot cereals and raisins |
| Scrambled-egg sandwich |

**Portable postworkout breakfasts**

These breakfasts contain carbohydrate and protein, perfect for postworkout.

| |
|---|
| Cereal bar and milk |
| Instant cereal and milk |
| Apple or banana, peanut butter, milk |
| Bagel with cream cheese |
| Hard-boiled egg with juice |
| Skim latté and a muffin |
| Yogurt and whole-grain crackers |
| Egg salad, turkey, or peanut butter sandwich and a bag of grapes |
| String cheese, apple, crackers |
| Graham crackers and peanut butter with milk |

## Fast Family Dinners

Athletes walk in the door after school practice sweaty, tired, and ravenous. They might find it nearly impossible to wait for dinner. If dinner isn't ready, they'll begin grazing through the kitchen, taking handfuls of cereal, crackers, and pretzels, chugging liquids right from the bottle, or standing in front of the refrigerator and eating last night's leftovers.

Parents can make this grazing time more manageable by having some good food ready for hungry athletes as they come in the door. A bowl of soup or salad or a roll with milk should be enough to tide them over until dinner is ready. Another strategy to reduce grazing is to teach your young athlete the importance of a recovery meal and ensure they pack a snack to eat right after practice.

Preparing dinner doesn't need to be a big production for the meal to be healthy. Enlist your children's help. Most cooks find three or four recipes and repeat them throughout the week. A five-day dinner rotation appears in table 9.3. Most of these meals lend themselves to reheating, and all of the recipes can be found in chapter 14.

**TABLE 9.2** Lunch in a Bag

| Protein foods (choose 1 or 2) | Grains (choose 1) | Veggies/fruit (choose 1, 2, or 3) | Dessert/snack (optional) | Beverages (choose 1) |
|---|---|---|---|---|
| Shaved lean meat | Bread | Celery | Chips/pretzels | 100% fruit juice |
| Hard-boiled or chopped eggs | Pita | Baby carrots | 2-3 cookies | Milk |
| Cheese cubes or string cheese | Bagel | Cucumber spears or coins | Frosted cereal | Water |
| Tuna fish | Tortilla | Green beans | Fruit/dessert yogurt | Seltzer water |
| Yogurt | Potato | Green beans | Pudding cup | |
| Cottage cheese | Rice | Melon, cubed or cut | Granola/ breakfast bar | |
| Chicken drum-stick | Pasta | Orange wedges | | |
| Peanut butter | Couscous | Kiwi slices | | |
| Hummus | English muffin | Berries | | |
| Beans, mashed or whole | Rolls | Pineapple cubes | | |
| Soup | | Applesauce | | |

Data: *Washington Parent Magazine.*


**TABLE 9.3** Mix-and-Match Dinners

Choose one from each column. (See recipes in chapter 14.)

| Protein | Grain | Veggie/fruit |
|---|---|---|
| Chicken breast stir fry | Rice | Frozen veggie stir fry |
| Ground turkey burger | Roll | Fruit salad |
| Fabulous flank steak | Potatoes | Frozen vegetables: broccoli, spinach |
| Skim milk | Pasta/tomato sauce | Salad bar veggies |
| Eggs | Bagel/toast | Spinach salad |
| Beans/ground beef | Flour tortilla | Lettuce/tomato/onions |
| Cheese | Pizza crust | Green salad |

## Sensible Snacking

Many parents admonish snacking for fear that it ruins appetites, but snacking is totally appropriate for children, particularly athletes. However, note the difference between snacking and grazing. Snacking, like meals, has a beginning and an end. Grazing is a continuous act of eating, often in a haphazard, impulsive way.

Snacks can be nutritious—or not. Grabbing something like cookies or chips as a snack isn't a great idea because most hungry kids will eat more than they should. Instead, think of snacks as mini-meals. A slice of pizza, a bowl of cereal with milk, or a cup of soup make great snacks. Foods that taste good but have little nutritious value (junk food) work better as desserts because you will be more likely to eat a reasonable amount than when eating them as snacks.

# Eating Game Plan

An athlete's training should include lessons about foods that are and aren't well tolerated before physical activity. Young athletes should understand the importance of fueling during events and eating immediately afterward to recover.

### Pregame Plan

Pregame meals are those meals eaten three to six hours before a game or other activity. The purpose of a pregame meal is to keep the blood sugar in a normal range and to add to the existing glycogen stores so that your athlete has a maximum amount of fuel before the event. The pregame meal should be well digested but filling enough for the athlete to avoid hunger during competition.

Normally, it takes about three to four hours to completely digest and absorb a regular mixed meal. As long as there's enough time for digestion, the pregame meal can be anything that contains carbohydrates, protein, and fat and which the athlete knows he or she can well tolerate (table 9.4).

Because fat takes longer to empty from the stomach, it's probably wise to avoid fried or high-fat foods on game day (and most other days). Eating high-fat foods can cause sluggishness because the energy they provide isn't as available as the energy from carbohydrate-rich food. Foods high in fiber, such as bran cereal, should also be avoided before exercise. Fiber can cause cramping as well as necessary bathroom visits at inconvenient times.

Athletes competing in events with short, intense bursts, such as sprinting, short-distance swimming, or rowing, should allow their stomachs to empty before competition starts to prevent nausea. During intense activity, working

**TABLE 9.4    Pregame Meals**

| Pregame guidelines |
| --- |
| Eat a pregame meal at least three hours before the game to allow for digestion. |
| Choose foods high in carbohydrates. Include moderate amounts of protein and fat, as tolerated. |
| Be sure the foods agree with you. Everyone has his or her own individual tolerance. |
| If you're nervous or jittery, a liquid meal might be a better choice. |
| Watch fiber content. You may not be able to tolerate foods high in fiber before an event. |
| Don't experiment on the day of a game. |
| Drink before, during, and after a game. |
| Choose foods you enjoy and you know make you feel good. |
| **Pregame breakfast (allow three hours to digest)** |
| Hot or cold cereal, milk, and fruit |
| Bagel with juice or milk |
| Muffins with milk or juice |
| Yogurt and toast |
| Frozen waffles or pancakes, juice, milk |
| **Pregame lunch/dinner (allow three hours to digest)** |
| Chicken or sliced turkey sandwich on whole-grain bread or roll, fruit or juice, milk |
| Pasta with tomato sauce, bread, fruit or juice, milk |
| Baked potato with cottage cheese and fruit or juice |
| Thick-crust pizza, fruit or juice |
| **Pregame snacks and liquid meals (eat within one to two hours before the game)** |
| Fruit |
| Sports bars or cereal bars and sports drink |
| Smoothie (fruit-based) |
| Dried cereal and juice |
| Dried fruit |

muscles channel blood flow away from the stomach, causing discomfort if exercise is begun with food still in the stomach.

For some athletes, eating a carbohydrate-rich snack within an hour before their event fuels them up. A piece of fruit, an energy bar, or some crackers should be easy to digest. Some athletes can tolerate anything they eat. Others find that drinking a carbohydrate drink such as juice is easier than eating. All of this depends wholly on the individual. Whatever athletes choose as their pregame meal should be familiar to their bodies and taste good. This is not a good time to experiment with new foods.

For early morning events, encourage athletes to get up early enough to allow time to eat. A carbohydrate-rich meal helps increase muscle glycogen before morning exercise. At the very least, have athletes drink a box drink of fruit juice and eat a cereal bar.

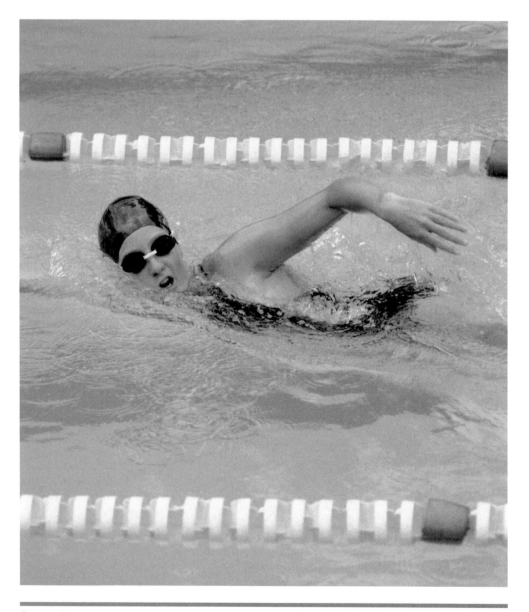

Short-distance swimmers should eat their premeet meal three to six hours before their event to avoid the nausea that can be caused by intense activity.

## During Events

Athletes know the phrase "hitting the wall" but usually associate it with distance runners depleting their glycogen stores and running out of gas.

**TABLE 9.5    Eating and Drinking on the Run**

Eat and drink during events to keep energy level high

- Sports drinks
- Fruit
- Sports bars

In fact, hitting the wall can happen in any sport. Soccer, football, and tennis use glycogen to fuel the intense stop-and-go activity common to these sports. Without snacking and drinking during these long games, athletes feel exhausted quickly and hit the wall.

When muscles are well nourished, with good glycogen stores at the beginning of an event, they perform longer if they also receive fuel during the event. Encourage athletes to take advantage of breaks in activity to eat or drink easy-to-digest, carbohydrate-rich foods such as fruit, energy bars, or sports drinks (tables 9.5 and 9.6). They'll feel more energetic throughout the event.

**TABLE 9.6    Comparing Sports Bars**

| Product | Calories | Protein | Carbohydrates | Fat | Comments |
|---|---|---|---|---|---|
| Balance® | 200 | 14 | 22 | 6 | Pre- and postworkout |
| Balance Gold® | 210 | 15 | 23 | 7 | Pre- and postworkout |
| Balance Outdoor® | 200 | 15 | 21 | 6 | Pre- and postworkout |
| Cliff® | 230 | 10 | 41 | 4 | Preworkout/endurance |
| Luna® | 180 | 10 | 25 | 4 | Pre- and postworkout |
| Met-Rx Food Bar® | 320 | 27 | 48 | 2.5 | Postworkout/meal |
| Odwalla® | 240 | 7 | 48 | 4 | Preworkout/short duration |
| PowerBar Harvest® | 240 | 7 | 45 | 4 | Preworkout/short duration |
| PowerBar Performance® | 230 | 10 | 45 | 3 | Preworkout/short duration |
| **In comparison** | | | | | |
| Nutrigrain® bar | 140 | 2 | 27 | 3 | Preworkout/short duration |
| Granola bar | 120 | 2 | 21 | 3 | Preworkout/short duration |
| Snickers® bar | 280 | 4 | 35 | 14 | |

Data: "Raising the Bar," December 2000, *Nutrition Action Healthletter*, and *Diets Designed for Athletes*, 27-30.

## Recovery

What you eat within the first few minutes after a workout or competition is known as your "recovery meal." This small meal is the most important and underrated part of training. It sets the stage for how the athlete feels for the rest of the day and affects the next day's training or competition.

Recovery eating is essentially reloading the muscles with glycogen. Fifteen to 30 minutes after exercising, the muscles are like sponges, waiting to refill the glycogen stores that have just been exhausted. If athletes refill within this time range, they'll be revved to go. If they miss their window of opportunity, they'll feel sluggish and lazy for the next event.

Carbohydrate plus protein appears to be the most effective combination for restoring glycogen. Eating a snack (such as a banana with yogurt) within 15 minutes of the end of a workout and then eating a regular meal 2 hours later maximizes muscle receptivity (table 9.7).

Many athletes just can't or don't want to eat directly after exercise. In such cases, drinking a sports drink or diluted fruit juice is a good first step to refueling. Athletes who want to lose weight often choose not to eat right after exercising; they rationalize that they've just burned a bunch of calories and shouldn't replace them right away. In fact, recovery eating often helps these athletes refrain from bingeing later in the day. Remember that the recovery meal is just a small eating episode—it's not breakfast, lunch, or dinner.

Planning meals for athletes is challenging, but the payoff makes it worthwhile. Young athletes feel much more energized if they take time for breakfast, lunch, and dinner. They'll have more productive workouts when they refuel correctly and can better manage their day. When families are involved in these meals, everyone benefits.

**TABLE 9.7     Eating to Recover**

This is reload food. Try to eat and drink within 15 minutes of exercising, and then again within an hour or two.

- Sports drink and trail mix with peanuts
- Mini-applesauce and peanut butter crackers
- Yogurt and fruit
- Graham crackers with peanut butter and juice
- Cereal bar with milk or juice
- Sports bar with water
- Fruit with string cheese and sports drink
- Mini-bagel with juice
- Turkey slices with juice
- Smoothie made with juice and protein powder

# Team Eating

Eating meals together is a great way for teams to bond. Most teams have ample opportunities to eat as a group. Some enjoy pregame meals together; others reward themselves with a stop at a special place immediately after a game to fuel up for recovery. Meals are also perfect times for coaches to show their athletes how much they value nutrition. Team meals should showcase the importance of eating well. Pregame team meals are often a time for traditional fare and favorite foods, but they can also be a chance to try something new.

---

## Team-Building Meals

Team meals can serve many purposes. They are an important tradition, an opportunity to boost team spirit and camaraderie, and of course an occasion for fueling the athletes. They are also an excellent chance to put good sports nutrition goals into practice. As coach, you might consider sending out a letter to team parents to gain their support for team meals. The letter could look something like this one:

Dear Team Parent:

The team meal is an important part of our team's tradition. We think it is an excellent way to boost team spirit and to show our athletes how much we value them. Because we believe team nutrition is an integral part of their training, please keep the following guidelines in mind when planning your meal:

- The meal should be eaten at least three hours before kick-off to allow plenty of time for digestion.
- The meal should include carbohydrate-rich foods such as pasta, bread, rolls, rice, or potatoes. Lean protein such as ground beef or ground poultry can also be included.
- Serve water with the meal.

---

# Talking to Your Athlete About Meal Planning

- Eating three meals a day plus snacks gives your athletes the energy they need for practice. Breakfast is especially important for athletes with early morning practice.

- Pregame meals should top off an already well-fueled tank. These meals should include only foods that the athletes tolerate well.

- It takes three to four hours to digest a regular meal. Light snacks digest within an hour.

- Athletes should avoid high-fat meals before exercising. High-fat food delays gastric emptying and makes athletes sluggish.

- Eat or drink a high-carbohydrate food during an event to keep energy level high.

- Recovery eating is essential to refuel muscles. A snack including protein and carbohydrate should be eaten 15 to 30 minutes after exercise to refuel properly.

# Chapter 10

# FAST-BREAK FOOD FAVORITES

Eating meals away from home was once reserved for special occasions. Now the typical family eats as many as 40 percent of their meals outside of the home. Restaurant eating is enjoyable and easy, and you avoid food battles among children because everyone can order what they like. However, the restaurant industry—especially those establishments that families frequent—plays into our love affair with salt, fat, sweet, and super-size. A steady diet of this sort of fare is bound to be detrimental, so we must take care to choose wisely.

Eating out is part of our culture. For many young people and families on the go, fast food best fits the lifestyle (even for those of us who are nutritionists). What's so appealing about fast food? Well, for one thing, it's fast. That in itself is very attractive to active families racing from one practice to another. Fast food is also predictable, and kids like familiarity. Although preparing a meal at home remains less expensive than eating fast food, occasional meals at McDonald's or Taco Bell won't break the bank.

Athletes and their families are going to find fast food at every turn. Sometimes it's the only choice, and sometimes it's the preferred choice. As adults, we're concerned about the long-term problems associated with the high-calorie, high-fat foods sold at fast-food restaurants. Most of our children don't share this concern. After all, kids are interested in how foods taste, not the toll they'll take on their bodies years from now. But unless we help them to make smart choices, the calories, fat, and sodium add up quickly for young athletes, too. They'll find that a steady diet of fast food is not the way to fuel for competition or sustained physical activity.

Danny, a growing 15-year-old, spent the summer playing junior golf. He rarely could eat on the course, although the average golf round lasted five to six hours. After exhausting, trying matches, often in hot, humid conditions, he left the tournaments famished. Fast food was always a short ride away. Because he was so hungry, he usually ordered too much and overate.

A steady postmatch diet of a Big Mac, large fries, and six chicken nuggets usually hit the spot for Danny. But after eight weeks of this, he was gaining weight. He decided to put a new plan into place. He began packing a peanut butter sandwich, a piece of fruit, and an energy bar to take out on the course. He always drank plenty of water or a sports drink. He ate the food slowly while walking from hole to hole. After the round was over, if he did choose to stop at a fast-food restaurant with friends, all he felt like having was a regular hamburger and water.

## Quick Doesn't Have to Mean Bad

One of the biggest problems with fast foods (and restaurants in general) is super-size meals. Restaurant portions tend to be huge. Entrees can be 8 to 12 ounces instead of the standard portion of 3 to 6 ounces. The super-size meal in a fast-food restaurant might look like a good deal, but it's always going to be more calories, more fat, and more food than one person needs at one time. If young athletes think they must order super-size meals to get their money's worth, encourage them to share the meals with friends or save some for later.

One of the most obvious examples of super-sizing is with beverages. At one time, a small drink at a fast-food place was 12 ounces. Now it's at least 16 ounces. Super-size drinks can contain as many as 400 calories. That's far more calories than anyone needs to drink with a meal. Often it's more than anyone *wants* to drink, but once the cup is in your hands, you end up finishing the whole thing. Encourage your young athletes to avoid the excess calories by choosing water, skim milk, or a small soft drink.

In fast-food restaurants, tell your youngsters to "go for plain." A plain burger is much healthier than a big specialty sandwich. Sauces added to burgers and sandwiches add flavor but at the cost of a lot of unnecessary fat and calories. Remind your children to request sauces and salad dressings on the side—then they can use them sparingly if they want them at all.

## Reading Menus

| This is a better choice . . . | Than this . . . |
| --- | --- |
| Roasted | Au gratin or cheese sauce |
| Steamed | Fried |
| Marinara sauce | Alfredo sauce |
| Grilled | Scampi style |
| Cooked in own juice | Cooked in butter, cream |
| Barbecued | Batter-dipped, tempura |
| Broiled | Breaded |
| Poached | Sautéed |
| Tomato sauce | Cream gravy |

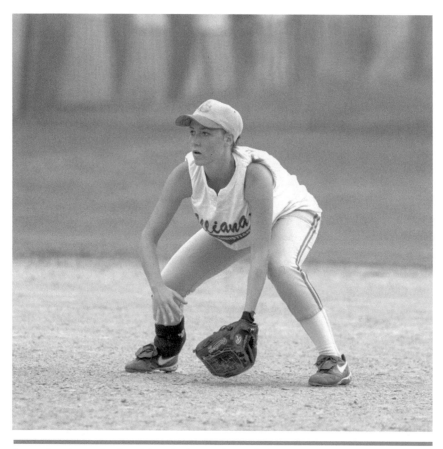

Learning to make healthy choices when dining out will help athletes perform their best on and off the field.

If the smaller burgers and sandwiches aren't filling enough to satisfy an active, growing child, improvise by making your own version of a double-decker sandwich. Order two plain sandwiches, such as a grilled chicken sandwich, a plain burger, or a plain cheeseburger. Take the patty from one and stack it on the other. This makes a filling, high-protein sandwich.

Some fast foods appear to be healthy but end up being nutritional nightmares. Teach your young athletes restaurant terminology so that they aren't fooled by foods that sound healthy but aren't. Fish, chicken, and salad bars all appear to be healthy additions to menus, but they must be chosen carefully. When fish and chicken are breaded and fried, they aren't any better than a high-fat burger. Order grilled sandwiches to get the healthier choice.

Salad bars can also be deceptive. If something grows in or on the ground, then it's properly placed on the salad bar. But if you're checking out a mayonnaise-laden salad or fried croutons or noodles, look the other way. These items on a salad bar add few nutrients and plenty of calories to what can otherwise be a healthy addition to meals (table 10.1).

**TABLE 10.1** Dissecting the Salad Bar

- Start with leafy greens such as lettuce and spinach.
- Pile high other fresh veggies, such as carrots, mushrooms, cucumbers, and peppers.
- Limit the prepared salads (pasta salad, marinated vegetable salad, potato salad).
- To make your salad an entrée rather than a side, add protein such as cottage cheese, eggs, tuna, cheese, chickpeas, tofu, or turkey.
- Skip the extras, such as croutons, bacon bits, and fried noodles.
- Dress the salad first with vinegar, salsa, or lemon; then add a small amount of olive oil or dressing of your choice.

| Veggies | Serving size | Calories | Fat | Protein |
|---|---|---|---|---|
| Artichoke hearts | ¼ cup | 18 | 0 | 1 |
| Bean sprouts | ¼ cup | 8 | 0 | 0 |
| Beets | ¼ cup | 20 | 0 | 0 |
| Broccoli | ½ cup | 12 | 0 | 1 |
| Cabbage | ½ cup | 8 | 0 | .5 |
| Carrots, shredded | ¼ cup | 15 | 0 | 0 |
| Cauliflower | ½ cup | 12 | 0 | 0 |
| Celery | ¼ cup | 5 | 0 | 0 |
| Corn | ¼ cup | 45 | .5 | 2.5 |
| Cucumbers | ¼ cup | 4 | 0 | 0 |
| Hearts of palm | ¼ cup | 10 | 0 | 1 |
| Lettuce | 1 cup | 12 | 0 | 0 |
| Mushrooms | ¼ cup | 5 | 0 | 0 |
| Onions | 1 tbsp | 4 | 0 | 0 |
| Peas | 2 tbsp | 30 | 0 | 0 |
| Peppers, red or green | 2 tbsp | 7 | 0 | 0 |
| Radishes | 2 tbsp | 2 | 0 | 0 |
| Spinach | 1 cup | 12 | 0 | 0 |
| Squash, yellow or green | ¼ cup | 5 | 0 | 0 |
| Tomatoes, chopped | ½ cup | 18 | 0 | 0 |
| **Protein choices** | | | | |
| Cheese, cottage (creamed) | ½ cup | 120 | 5 | 14 |
| Cheese, cottage (low-fat) | ½ cup | 80 | 2 | 12 |
| Cheese, grated parmesan | 2 tbsp | 45 | 3 | 4 |
| Cheese, shredded cheddar | 3 tbsp | 115 | 10 | 7 |
| Chickpeas | ½ cup | 120 | 2 | 7 |
| Eggs, chopped | 2 tbsp | 25 | 2 | 7 |
| Tofu | ½ cup | 94 | 6 | 10 |
| Tuna, plain | 2 tbsp | 60 | 1 | 13 |
| Turkey, diced | 2 tbsp | 60 | 1.5 | 10 |

## Prepared Salads

| | | | | |
|---|---|---|---|---|
| Carrot raisin | ¼ cup | 105 | 7 | 6 |
| Macaroni | ½ cup | 135 | 5 | 3 |
| Marinated artichoke | ¼ cup | 41 | 3 | 1 |
| Pasta | ½ cup | 150 | 8 | 2.5 |
| Potato | ½ cup | 179 | 10 | 3 |
| Three bean | ½ cup | 7 | 4 | 2 |
| Tuna | ¼ cup | 96 | 5 | 8 |
| Waldorf (apples, nuts) | ½ cup | 48 | 3 | .5 |
| **Extras** | | | | |
| Bacon bits | 1 tbsp | 25 | 1.5 | 2 |
| Chow mein noodles | 2 tbsp | 150 | 9 | 2 |
| Croutons | 2 tbsp | 50 | 2 | 1 |
| Olives | 5 large | 25 | 2 | 0 |
| Pickles | 1 medium | 5 | 0 | 0 |
| Raisins | 1 tbsp | 60 | 0 | 0 |
| Sunflower seeds | 2 tbsp | 180 | 16 | 7 |
| **Dressings\*** | | | | |
| Bleu cheese | 2 tbsp | 160 | 16 | 1 |
| Bleu cheese, fat-free | 2 tbsp | 36 | 0 | 0 |
| Caesar | 2 tbsp | 158 | 17 | 0 |
| Caesar, fat-free | 2 tbsp | 30 | 0 | 0 |
| French | 2 tbsp | 130 | 11 | 0 |
| French, fat-free | 2 tbsp | 43 | 1 | 0 |
| Italian | 2 tbsp | 140 | 15 | 0 |
| Ranch | 2 tbsp | 180 | 20 | 0 |
| Ranch, fat-free | 2 tbsp | 34 | 0 | 0 |
| Salsa | 2 tbsp | 8 | 0 | 0 |
| Soy sauce | 2 tbsp | 10 | 0 | 0 |
| Thousand Island | 2 tbsp | 160 | 16 | 0 |
| Thousand Island, fat-free | 2 tbsp | 50 | 0 | 0 |
| Vinegar | 2 tbsp | 4 | 0 | 0 |

\*1 ladle of dressing at a salad bar = 4 tbsp

Adapted, by permission, from A. Litt, 2000, *The College Student's Guide to Eating Well on Campus*, (Bethesda, MD: Tulip Hill), 41-42.

Watch out for the "extras" on the menu or that are brought to the table in a restaurant. A bowl of noodles in a Chinese restaurant or a bread basket placed in front of a hungry group is hard to resist. Having these foods with a meal is fine, but filling up on them before a meal is served leads to overeating. The same is true with sides such as hushpuppies, biscuits, buttered bread sticks, and fries—all are tasty but loaded with calories, and if you fill up on them, you end up too full to enjoy your main course. Have the side dishes occasionally rather than always.

Fast-food restaurants do have some excellent choices, including skim milk, garden salads, and soups. See table 10.2 for smart fast-food choices. In a sit-down restaurant, fresh fruit is usually available (though not always on the menu). If you eat out frequently, be sure to include fruit, vegetables, and salads with your meals.

### TABLE 10.2    Choosing Better Fast Food

Avoid unnecessary calories and fat by making smarter choices when eating fast food.

| Choose this . . . | | Instead of this . . . | |
|---|---|---|---|
| | (Calories/fat/protein) | | (Calories/fat/protein) |
| **McDonald's** | | | |
| ¼-pounder | (430/21/23) | Big Mac | (590/34/24) |
| Medium fries | (450/22/6) | Super-size fries | (610/29/9) |
| Water | (0) | Large soda | (350) |
| *Total meal* | 880/43/29 | | 1550/63/33 |
| McGrill | (300/6/24) | Crispy chicken | (500/26/22) |
| Small fries | (210/10/3) | Large fries | (540/26/8) |
| Milk | (100/2.5/8) | Vanilla shake | (570/16/14) |
| *Total meal* | (610/18.5/35) | | (1610/68/44) |
| **Pizza Hut** | | | |
| 2 slices hand-tossed pizza | (480/20/24) | 2 slices New York-style pizza | (820/36/40) |
| **Taco Bell** | | | |
| 2 chicken soft tacos | (380/12/28) | 2 double-deck tacos | (680/28/30) |
| **Chinese food** | | | |
| Broccoli and beef, steamed rice | (563/18/19) | Orange chicken, lo mein | (895/35/39) |
| **Subway** | | | |
| 6-inch roast beef sub | (303/5/20) | 6-inch tuna sub | (542/32/29) |

One of the more appealing aspects of fast food is that it is fast. Eating too fast, however, can lead to overeating. Try to slow down when you're eating. Stop eating before you feel full. Chew slowly and savor each bite. If you're at a restaurant, have uneaten food removed promptly so that you don't pick at it until it's gone.

If your dining-out experience is only once in a while, go ahead and go all out. Eat whatever you want. Perhaps an occasional disregard for good nutrition is good for the soul. But if you eat out often, make a plan and stick to it. Choose healthy meals, even at fast-food restaurants. It can be done. It just takes commitment and planning.

---

## Talking to Your Athlete About Eating Out

- Pay attention to super-sizing. Super-size means you're going to eat more than you need. If you think super-size meals are a bargain, split them with a friend.
- Build a better burger. Stay away from big burger-type sandwiches. Order plain and add your own toppings.
- Don't be fooled by fish and fowl. Breaded and fried fish, chicken, and nuggets are not necessarily healthier choices than burgers. A tuna fish sandwich made with oil-packed tuna rather than water-packed can have as much fat and as many calories as a Big Mac.
- Order the extras that count. Low-fat and fat-free milk, salads, soups, and fruit are good additions to a meal away from home.
- Drink carefully. Avoid large sodas and shakes unless you're trying to gain weight. Instead order water or low-fat milk.

# Chapter 11

# BEYOND THE STANDARD GAME PLAN WITH SUPPLEMENTS

The supplement industry knows their market. As many as 50 percent of high school athletes admit to using supplements at some point. With more than 29,000 supplements to choose from and millions of dollars spent advertising them, it's a challenge to determine whether they're helpful or unnecessary, legal or banned, safe or harmful.

All athletes are looking for a competitive edge. Can they find it in a drink, pill, or potion? Unlikely. Will they be tempted to try? Absolutely. Before they spend one penny or, worse, put themselves at risk by doing something harmful or illegal, they better know the facts.

Supplements are targeted at athletes to improve their performance. Testimonials and endorsements make them hard to resist. It's difficult to dismiss claims laced with scientific-sounding support (though it's often taken out of context). All of this makes supplements very appealing for some athletes. They are easy to get and easy to use. Let's face it—they are very seductive, especially to risk-taking teens.

## What Are Supplements?

Ergogenic, or "work-producing," supplements are promoted to athletes as substances that they need in larger amounts than the typical diet supplies. They include many products marketed to athletes for the specific purpose of improving performance. Claimed benefits to athletes include

- increased muscle size,

- greater strength,
- improved endurance,
- better speed, and
- improved weight loss through fat burning.

Looking over this list, nearly any athlete would be tempted to try a supplement. Even some coaches might prove susceptible to the lure. But smart coaches don't buy the hype. There are problems with testing, quality, legality, safety, and long-term effects that should always be a concern to anyone considering using supplements.

The American Academy of Pediatrics feels that high-performance supplements have no place in the diets of young children. Though this is true, it's important when your athletes are discussing supplements not to dismiss their use by saying something like, "This isn't good for you; you shouldn't use it." Instead, tell them about the lack of scientific evidence for the use of supplements, the lack of standards governing what's in them, and the fact that some might contain ingredients deemed illegal by sports organizations.

As a coach or parent, it's your job to know what your athletes are taking by asking questions and observing. Vitamins and minerals, amino acids, protein powders, and even energy bars are considered supplements. Young athletes might be surprised to know that popular sports drinks are also considered supplements. Surely there are safe and useful supplements, then?

Don't assume anything when it comes to supplements. Certain supplements, such as sports drinks, are generally safe to use. Some, however, might have added ingredients that are not safe or legal for athletes. Coaches and parents should explain to young athletes that some of the supplements they can purchase might be banned by governing organizations, including the NCAA. If a seemingly safe product contains an ingredient that is unsafe or illegal and your athletes use it, they are in trouble. The "I didn't know" defense doesn't work. For a complete list of substances banned by the NCAA, visit the NCAA Web site at www.NCAA.org.

The supplement issue gets very murky because some supplements actually show promise, but they have not been tested on growing children. What might be safe for adults might not be safe for children. To encourage children to use supplements without knowing their long-term safety is grossly irresponsible.

## What You See Is Not Always What You Get

Supplements are virtually unregulated. They are not considered food or drugs, which means the Food and Drug Administration (FDA), the government watchdog agency responsible for regulating food and drugs, doesn't regulate them. In fact, no one regulates anything related to supplements. Basically, it's buyer beware. We are all fair game for marketing scams, unscientific claims, poor quality control, and, if we purchase a product, possible injury. That's pretty scary when you realize that your impressionable 13-year-old, grasping at anything to become bigger, faster, or stronger, can walk into a store and purchase what is essentially a drug. Young athletes may not have the savvy to evaluate the claims made. They may be unaware of how the product interacts with other substances, some of which can be potentially deadly combinations. And if they're like most kids, they might think if some is good, more is better.

---

Joey, a 16-year-old football player, decided that he needed to get bigger. He walked into the local health food store and, with guidance from the clerk, purchased several supplements marketed as muscle builders.

What Joey didn't know was that taking all of these supplements at once was not a good idea. Nothing on the label indicated that a combination of these supplements with other drugs or supplements could be harmful.

Joey started taking the supplements and immediately saw an increase in his muscle mass. One day, about two weeks into using the supplements, he was in the workout room at school. Joey had a seizure caused by combining certain chemicals found in the supplements he had been taking. He was rushed to a hospital, where he remained in intensive care for 10 days.

Today, Joey is a capable football player who eats well and trains correctly and will never use supplements again.

---

Quality control is a huge issue with supplements. They can contain the ingredients listed on the label—or not. They might contain substances not listed on the label, a potential problem for anyone with allergies. It's also possible that you might not actually be purchasing what you think you are. Claims made for supplements range from accurate to totally false. Some have been well researched; others have not. Evaluating the many claims is difficult. Two Web sites—www.supplementwatch.com and www.consumerlab.com—offer information from independent testing laboratories and provide unbiased information about supplements (table 11.1).

With all that is wrong with supplements, it's also true that some are harmless. Some may have produced encouraging results but have never been tested on children. Most are expensive and not at all needed. As a coach or parent of a young athlete, you need to know about the popular supplements so that you can provide information to your athlete.

**TABLE 11.1    Evaluating Claims About Supplements**

| |
|---|
| • If it sounds too good to be true, it is. |
| • Testimonials are convincing, but they are not scientific. |
| • Recognize the placebo effect. In many cases, just believing something will help yield results. |
| • Ask for the qualifications of the person recommending the product. Does he or she profit by selling it to you? |
| • Watch for buzz words and phrases such as secret formula, detoxify, energize, miraculous results. |

# Popular Supplements

This section takes a look at some of the supplements often discussed among teenage athletes. The list is by no means comprehensive but provides a peek at what your athletes might be thinking about.

## Amino Acids and Protein Powders

*Claims:* Amino acids, the building blocks of protein, are needed in larger amounts than the diet provides because athletes have higher protein needs than the general population. Protein powders found in drinks and supplements are superior to those naturally found in food sources. Amino acids such as the branched chain amino acids (BCAA) reportedly increase the release of human growth hormone, which is responsible for promoting muscle growth and increasing strength.

*Facts:* Athletes do have higher protein needs than nonathletes, but it's quite possible to meet protein needs through food sources. Both BCAA and other proteins are plentiful in the typical diet. When taking individual amino acids, you run the risk of creating an imbalance in your body's amino acid pool.

Protein powder supplements can be quite expensive. While using them isn't necessary, they probably belong on the list of supplements that aren't harmful to use as long as the labeling is accurate and they don't contain any additional ingredients.

## Vitamins and Minerals

*Claims:* Vitamins and minerals are necessary for properly metabolizing and digesting all food eaten. They give you energy. More is better. Since athletes need more food than nonathletes do, it makes sense that they would need more vitamins and minerals.

*Facts:* Most people don't think of vitamins and minerals as supplements, but they are categorized that way. Vitamins and minerals are naturally present in many foods. Athletes eat more food than other people, so they should be able to get the vitamins and minerals they need without taking a supplement. Vitamins and minerals do not contain calories, so they don't supply energy. They act as sparkplugs and help ensure that calories are used properly.

Supplements can be helpful in some situations (table 11.2). For instance, athletes who can't tolerate dairy products can get the calcium they need by taking supplements. Athletes who follow a strict vegetarian diet are often advised to find foods with added vitamin B$_{12}$. But of course these aren't the arguments that athletes hear for using supplements.

## Table 11.2    Choosing a Vitamin or Mineral Supplement

**You don't get what you pay for.** Natural or synthetic generally doesn't matter, because your body can't recognize whether the supplement was manufactured in a lab or came from a natural source. For most supplements, it doesn't matter whether you buy a store brand, name brand, or natural. The only differences might be the ingredients added for taste, the packaging, and the price.

**Check the expiration date.** Vitamins lose their potency, so buy the one with the longest shelf life.

**One hundred percent is enough.** Because it's possible to get toxic amounts of some vitamins and minerals, play it safe and stay with those that contain about 100 percent of the standard. More is not better and can be unsafe for vitamin A, calcium, folic acid, or vitamin D.

**Choose a vitamin–mineral combo.** That way you can avoid disturbing the delicate balance that makes vitamins and minerals work best. In certain situations, you might need more than a standard supplement provides.

**Timing is important.** It's best to take your supplement with meals. If you're taking a multivitamin with iron, don't take extra calcium at the same time because each is absorbed better when taken separately.

**Food first.** All of the expensive supplements in the store won't replace a healthy diet.

Adapted, by permission, from A. Litt, 2000, *The College Student's Guide to Eating Well on Campus*, (Bethesda, MD: Tulip Hill), 23.

## Creatine

*Claims:* Creatine increases muscle mass and lean body mass, allowing athletes to train more. It speeds recovery time during intense activity so is helpful for athletes involved in such sports as football, hockey, and soccer. *Facts:* Creatine is by far the most popular supplement used today. It is an amino acid compound synthesized in the body and found in high-protein foods such as meat and fish. Supplementing with creatine does in fact increase strength and body mass in some athletes. The response varies considerably from athlete to athlete.

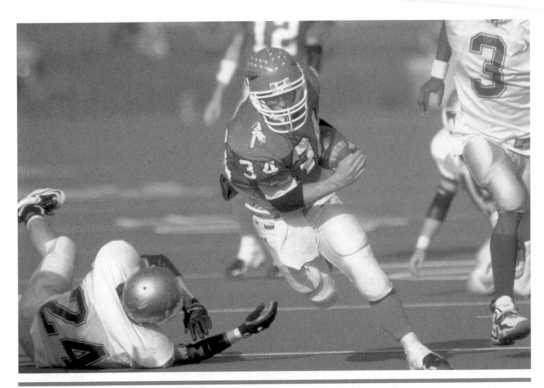

Despite the lack of studies on long-term effects, a football player may be tempted to use creatine to increase muscle mass and improve recovery time during the game's intense activity.

Reported side effects with the use of creatine include weight gain and cramping. Its benefits decrease when supplementation is discontinued. Poor quality control is a problem because the amount and purity of the supplement being purchased isn't reliable. Dosing is an issue and must be done carefully. More creatine is not better.

Creatine use has never been studied in athletes who are still growing. Because its long-term effects on growing bodies are unknown, creatine supplementation for a growing athlete is not recommended.

## DHEA and Androstenedione

*Claims:* DHEA and other prohormones, such as androstenedione (andro), are precursors to testosterone and increase energy, strength, and muscle development. They decrease recovery time, allowing harder training and better results.

*Facts:* Home-run hero Mark McGwire popularized andro, and both DHEA and andro are very popular supplements with teenagers. There's no scientific support for the claims that they increase strength and muscle mass.

Reported side effects include increased breast development, lowered libido in men, and stunted growth in children. Although DHEA and andro are legal to buy, they have the potential to raise testosterone and are considered a testosterone precursor that is banned by the International Olympic Committee, NCAA, and other governing bodies. Athletes using these supplements have failed doping tests. These supplements should never be recommended to growing athletes.

## Caffeine

*Claims:* Caffeine can help athletes participating in endurance sports by allowing them to go for a longer time without feeling exhausted. Caffeine helps athletes stay focused.

*Facts:* Caffeine has been around for centuries. Its effect on athletic performance varies from athlete to athlete. Some athletes report a clearer, stronger focus; others say they feel jittery and distracted after taking caffeine.

The NCAA bans caffeine in large doses. It has never been tested on growing athletes and should not be recommended as a supplement for them.

## Meal Replacements

*Claims:* Meal replacements are complete meals, balanced perfectly for athletes. The mix contains the precise type and amount of protein and vitamins and minerals that athletes need.

*Facts:* Although they should never replace a full meal, these meals do offer convenience to an athlete on the go. They are an expensive alternative to some of the blender drinks but easy to use. Be sure to check ingredients carefully because some meal replacements contain ergogenic substances such as ephedrine and creatine.

## Ephedra

*Claims:* A natural product, ephedra effectively speeds weight loss. It's found in products such as Ripped Fuel, Xenadrine, Ultimate Orange, and Hydroxycut, all marketed as fat burners.

*Facts:* Just because ephedra (ma huang) is from an herb, that does not make it safe. In fact, when coupled with other products (caffeine, aspirin) or when taken in large amounts, it can be deadly. Natural or not, ephedra is unsafe and illegal to use in many sports. Side effects of ephedra range from minor complaints of stomach discomfort and dizziness to serious problems such as high blood pressure, seizures, and death. Most recently, ephedra has been implicated in the death of 23-year-old Baltimore Orioles pitcher Steve Bechler. The IOC and the NCAA have banned it. Ephedra is definitely not to be recommended to young athletes.

## Functional Foods

*Claims:* There are various claims about functional foods, depending on the ingredients added to products. These foods are generally seen as "magic bullets" to enhance performance and recovery, increase weight loss, and add energy.

*Facts:* Functional foods are defined by the American Dietetic Association as "usually understood to be any potentially healthful food or food ingredient that may provide a health benefit beyond the traditional nutrients it contains." Examples of functional foods for athletes include designer waters with vitamins added, smoothies with additional protein, and sports bars with lycopene. The term *functional* implies that the food has some identified value leading to health benefits, including reduced risk for disease, for the person consuming it.

Like all other supplements, functional foods should be evaluated with a focus on safety and legality. Functional foods should never be used in place of healthy foods but might sometimes be appropriate in addition to a healthy diet.

## Guiding Athletes

Until supplements are regulated, issues about quality control, false claims, and safety will endure. The children you're coaching today may be coaching their own children before we have any good data on which, if any, supplements work and are safe for the growing athlete. Although some supplements appear to be safe, they never replace a healthy diet and a good training program.

As a coach or parent, you have the privilege of influencing a child's life. Teaching young athletes the importance of proper hydration, good nutrition, and a great training program to help them become better athletes is an important part of their development. To condone the use of supplements when their safety is questionable not only puts the young athletes at risk but also sends a message that winning must occur, no matter the costs.

## Talking to Your Athlete About Supplements

- Supplements are unregulated. You can never be sure what's in the product you're purchasing and if it's safe or effective.

- Dietary supplements are not recommended for children. Most supplements appear to be unnecessary. Those that show promise have never been tested on children.

- Taking a vitamin–mineral supplement is only helpful when a diet is deficient. Extra vitamins and minerals in an already adequate diet aren't going to make a difference.

- Some supplements, such as sports drinks and meal replacements, might be helpful in addition to eating a good diet.

- Training and eating well, not taking supplements, are what make a winner.

# Chapter 12

# SPECIAL NUTRITIONAL NEEDS FOR PREADOLESCENT ATHLETES

Children are playing organized sports at much younger ages than ever before. Selecting a sport, training year-round, and competing at an elite level are becoming increasingly common for preadolescents. This trend raises concern for those who worry about the effects of injuries from repetitive use, the psychological ramifications of intense competition at a young age, and the logistics of propelling a growing body through an exhausting schedule at the expense of other normal childhood activities.

Because of the importance of eating a diet adequate for growth, development, and performance, feeding preteen athletes presents unique challenges. Younger athletes are not mini-versions of teenage athletes. They have different nutritional needs that can't be quantified easily because of the wide-ranging growth rates that occur in this age group and the limited research available on nutrient requirements for young people.

## Nutrients for Growing Athletes

The increased need for nutrients for the growing athlete coupled with concerns about training and coping with changing bodies makes nutrition a particularly important issue for coaches and parents.

## Calories

Younger children are less efficient in moving their bodies. Because of their relative lack of coordination, they tend to waste calories. Partly for this reason, we shouldn't use adult formulas to determine the caloric needs of the child athlete. The best way to determine whether children are getting enough calories is to observe their growth and energy levels. If they are growing as is predicted for their own specific growth curve, they are probably eating enough to meet their needs.

Young, active children who eat the right amount may still appear tired. We should assess their entire schedule before jumping to the conclusion that inadequate nutrition is the culprit. Although it's tempting to bribe or cajole a child to eat more food, it's usually best to let the child determine how much is enough. Rather than forcing a child to eat more, parents can be most helpful to the young growing athlete by sticking to consistent meal patterns in which adequate and acceptable foods are offered at scheduled times in a stress-free environment.

## Protein

The younger the child, the higher his or her protein needs per unit of body weight (table 12.1). Even with increased protein needed by the younger athlete, it's still quite easy to meet protein requirements through eating a well-balanced diet. Children often prefer lower-quality protein sources such as chicken nuggets, luncheon meats, and hot dogs, but try to include a good source of protein at each meal, even if it's a glass of milk, a bagel with peanut butter instead of margarine, or yogurt for dessert.

A young child on a vegetarian diet can be well nourished (see chapter 4). Parents should not panic if their child proclaims one night at the dinner table that he or she will eat no more meat. Use the opportunity to offer the child some nutrition counseling. If the child is serious about becoming vegetarian and sticks with it for several weeks, you might want to consult a registered dietitian for guidance on developing healthy eating patterns for the child.

**TABLE 12.1    Protein Requirements for Younger Children***

| Age | Protein requirement |
| --- | --- |
| 7-10 years | 1.1-1.2 gm/kg/day |
| 11-14 years | 1.0 gm/kg/day |
| Adult | 0.8-1.0 gm/kg/day |

* This table contains protein requirements for children and does not consider the additional protein required by the young athlete (see chapter 4).

## Fluid

Young and active children must take in plenty of fluids. They are more likely than older children to become dehydrated. Young athletes produce more metabolic heat during exercise and don't sweat as easily as adults, so their cooling systems don't work as efficiently. Plus, young children are less likely to drink, even when fluids are available. They simply don't think of it. Remind all young children to drink before, during, and after practices and games; watch them to make sure they do so.

Young children do not tolerate temperature extremes; it takes them more time to acclimatize to changes in the environment. When starting new seasons, especially in extreme weather, proceed much more slowly with young children to allow them to adjust to the climate.

Pay special attention to obese children who start exercising. They require more effort than other children to do the same activity. Consequently, their temperature can rise faster than expected. Encourage them to stop frequently for fluid and rest, always being extremely careful not to sound as if you're singling them out because of their size.

## Minerals

For the young athlete, everything is forming and growing in the body. Bone health is particularly important. Research shows that many young athletes have inadequate calcium intake, possibly because they are concerned with the calories and fat dairy products provide.

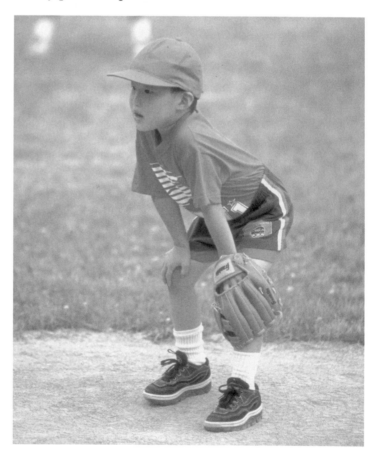

Young athletes need adequate amounts of calcium and iron for their growing bodies.

Adequate calcium intake is not only essential for normal bone formation but possibly reduces the risk of fractures and accelerates the healing process of broken bones. Encouraging sufficient calcium intake for young athletes is a high nutrition priority. Good sources of calcium are listed in table 4.3 (page 39).

Iron needs are extremely high at this stage in growth. In addition to the iron required for the formation of hemoglobin, training can increase iron loss from the body. Iron-rich foods might be limited, especially if the child has eliminated meat from the diet. Iron needs can be met in a vegetarian diet, but parents and coaches must ensure the child is eating adequate nonmeat sources of iron. Table 4.3 (page 39) lists good sources of iron for growing young athletes.

# Body Changes

The body of a prepubescent is not the same body of the child after puberty. When thinness is important in a sport, athletes may become highly competent before their bodies go through puberty. As the body fleshes out for puberty, they may get discouraged because their new bodies aren't as desirable for their sport and they're not achieving the same level of success.

As the body starts changing, some young athletes search for anything they can do to reverse the anticipated, perhaps dreaded, changes. This is one reason prepubescent athletes are at risk for developing eating disorders. Research shows that athletes with eating disorders begin specializing in sports significantly earlier than athletes who don't develop eating disorders.

The adolescent boy who goes through puberty early and grows tall faster than his peers might have to accept that his height at 12 years old is not enough to help him make his high school basketball team. At the opposite end of the spectrum, a late-blooming teenage boy might have played lacrosse as a preteen, but as his friends went through puberty they left him and his undeveloped body on the sidelines because he had not yet grown.

Body changes can be devastating. Even children who are laid back and tend to go with the flow can be significantly influenced by change to their bodies, particularly if their "new" body looks different from the bodies of their friends. For revved-up, intense, supersensitive young athletes, body changes can be even harder to adjust to. The years between 9 and 12 are especially sensitive ages for children. Coaches and parents can help by learning and appreciating the growth patterns and stages of development of prepubescents so that they're prepared to help children cope with normal body changes.

# Working With Younger Kids

The optimal diet for the young child isn't much different from that for anyone else. The main difference is that parents are more in charge and should use that to their advantage. The parents' job is to buy the proper foods, prepare them well, and establish age-appropriate times for meals and snacks. Parents should also spell out what is and isn't acceptable eating behavior in their homes and recognize the need for structure around mealtimes, especially for younger children.

Coaches, remember that practices must adhere to realistic time schedules so that your young athletes get plenty of rest and can eat properly. Without scheduled breaks for snacks and fluids, younger kids may forget to eat and drink and will consequently lose focus. Schedule frequent fluid breaks and encourage good snacks before and after practice. Give parents guidelines for the snacks they or their children bring to games.

Parents, stay involved! Be great role models for your children by eating and drinking properly. Watch their habits and patterns; communicate clearly if you see anything unusual.

---

## Snacking at Games

Providing snacks is a great way to build team-eating goals. Suggest that the team pitch in at the beginning of the season to invest in a few large coolers. During games and even practices, the coolers can be stocked with ice to keep beverages, yogurt, and fruit cold. Snacks during games should be mainly fluids (water and sports drinks) and cut-up fruit such as oranges and watermelon, especially in the summer. Post-training snacks should be carbohydrate-rich foods such as fruits, bagels, or small boxes of cereal. Also have some small protein foods handy, such as string cheese, yogurt, or peanut butter on graham crackers. Though junk foods are okay for growing athletes to eat now and then, it's wise to teach them the benefit of refueling properly.

---

Although young athletes are capable of eating well, their capacity for using nutrition information is limited. When working with this age group, coaches and parents will want to decide how much nutrition information their kids should receive, how much they can and should incorporate, and how much is too much for the child to handle.

These are critical years for forming good habits; you don't want to miss the opportunity to help your children develop healthy eating habits. But do so with balance, variety, and moderation in mind. Young children aren't all that interested in the role that food plays in their bodies. They are interested in what tastes good, what fills them when they are hungry, and what gives them energy to keep going.

Working with children is always a balancing act. Make sure your kids get the right amount of nutrients, but don't turn them into science projects. They are young and growing and have tremendous needs, but filling these needs is our opportunity to influence habits that can last a lifetime.

## Talking to Your Athlete About Nutritional Needs

- Younger athletes have varying growth rates and nutritional needs. Be sure children eat enough to allow them to grow normally and have the energy they need to participate in activities.
- To encourage proper hydration, coaches should develop practice schedules that make time for frequent fluid breaks.
- Parents have a tremendous opportunity to model good eating behaviors by planning nutritious meals and snacks and scheduling meal and snack times.
- Children have higher protein needs that *can* be met through food sources. Because they often prefer lower-quality protein, always offer good sources of acceptable protein at meals.
- Remind young children that their changing bodies are normal. The body they have at this age should be viewed as a beautiful work in progress.

# Chapter 13

# STRATEGIES FOR OVERCOMING DISORDERED EATING

Driven, coachable, hard working—these are among the qualities that define successful athletes. Unfortunately, they are the same traits that increase an athlete's risk of developing eating disorders. These personality traits along with a culture obsessed with appearance and the knowledge that eating well affects performance put a lot of pressure on a competitive young athlete. The good news is that not every athlete who is concerned about food and weight is eating disordered. So, as a parent or coach, how can you tell the difference?

## Spotting an Eating Disorder

Eating disorders are complex psychosocial problems characterized by obsessions about weight, food, and body image. On the surface, they are glamorized and trendy and often appear benign. Unfortunately, they can have serious, irreversible effects on health and body functions. They can be psychologically devastating. And in severe cases they can result in death.

Eating disorders are diagnosed and classified by a specific set of criteria established by the *Diagnostic and Statistical Manual of Mental Disorders* (DSM). There are four diagnosable eating disorders: anorexia nervosa, bulimia, binge-eating disorders, and disordered eating (or anorexia athletica).

*Anorexia nervosa* is characterized by an overwhelming fear of being fat, weight loss, a refusal to maintain an acceptable weight, and a preoccupation with food. On the surface, anorexia appears to be a diet gone crazy, but there's a much deeper and disturbing component to it.

## Signs and Symptoms of Anorexia Nervosa

- Weight loss leading to a body weight of 85 percent of what's considered acceptable
- Intense fear of being fat or gaining weight
- Disturbed body image—feels fat in spite of extremely low weight
- Frequent weighing
- Denial of hunger
- Ritualistic eating habits, such as cutting food into tiny pieces, eating alone, and dragging out meals
- Loss of menstrual period
- Excessive exercise
- Rigidity about food and meals
- Creating list of foods not liked or avoided for "legitimate" reasons (such as being a vegetarian or being lactose intolerant)
- Perfectionist
- Preoccupation with food—cooks and prepares food for others, involved in food-related work, watches food shows, reads recipes constantly
- Increased sensitivity to cold
- Refusal to admit eating patterns are abnormal
- Social withdrawal

*Bulimia* is characterized by the uncontrolled eating of large amounts of food and then compensating by purging to get rid of it. Purging can take the form of induced vomiting, taking laxatives or diuretics, or overexercising.

## Signs and Symptoms of Bulimia

- Preoccupation with food, weight, and appearance
- Ingesting large volumes of food and then "getting rid" of it through vomiting, fasting, exercising, or taking laxatives
- Making excuses to go to the bathroom after eating
- Usually near a normal weight but with weight fluctuations
- Mood swings and depression
- Dental problems
- Stomach and digestive problems, such as bloating, constipation, diarrhea
- Scratched or scarred knuckles from scraping against teeth to induce vomiting
- Irritation of the esophagus and throat
- Low self-esteem

- Realization that eating pattern is abnormal
- Constant feelings of hunger
- Irregular menstrual periods
- Lightheadedness and headaches

*Binge-eating disorder* is characterized by reoccurring episodes of bingeing without purging.

## Signs and Symptoms of Binge-Eating Disorder
- Weight gain or obesity
- Stomach and digestive problems
- Quick eating
- Eating when not physically hungry or binge eating
- Preoccupation with eating, dieting, and weight
- Frequent dieting without losing weight
- Eating to escape problems and emotions
- Eating "normally" or "dieting" with others, then eating large amounts of food when alone
- Eating to the point of feeling uncomfortably full
- Feelings of guilt or depression after a binge
- Low self-esteem
- Realization that eating pattern is abnormal

Adapted, by permission, from A. Litt, 2000, *The College Student's Guide to Eating Well on Campus*, (Bethesda, MD: Tulip Hill), 108, 112, 113.

*Eating disorder,* not otherwise specified, is more commonly referred to as *disordered eating.* This problem involves a pattern of eating behaviors rather than a specific eating disorder. These individuals may not meet all the established criteria to be diagnosed clinically as having a full-blown eating disorder, but their conditions can be every bit as serious. The term *anorexia athletica* is often used for athletes who show signs of eating disorders but do not meet the established criteria for having one. For the coach, parent, and health care provider, this category poses the greatest challenge.

## Signs and Symptoms of Anorexia Athletica
- Compulsive exercise
- Amenorrhea
- Restrictive eating
- Intense fear of weight gain and getting fat even when very lean
- Occasional bingeing and purging to control weight

## At-Risk Athletes

Eating disorders occur in any sport and at any level of competition but tend to be most prevalent in three categories of sports:

- Weight-classification sports, such as wrestling and lightweight crew
- Sports where leanness enhances performance, such as distance running
- Aesthetic sports where bodies are judged, such as gymnastics and diving

Athletes, especially females, are more vulnerable to developing eating disorders than are other members of the general population. They are part of a teen culture where being thin is being in. Teenage girls often engage in body bashing as a way of bonding. Words like *anorexic* and *bulimic* are part of their vocabulary, allowing these insidious disorders to leak into the mainstream.

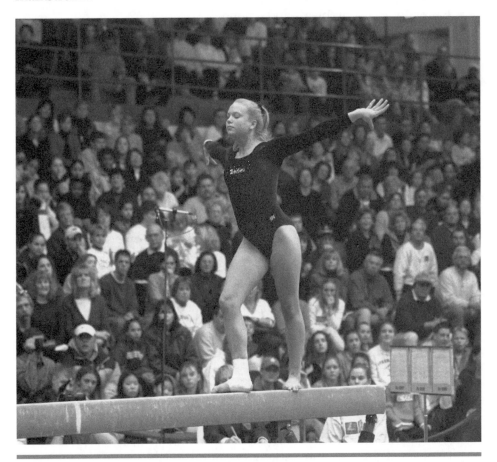

Girls face a pressure to be thin, especially in an aesthetic sport like gymnastics.

Like all children, young female athletes are bombarded daily by media that promotes ultrathin bodies as normal and ideal. Many celebrities meet the diagnostic criteria for having an eating disorder, but young girls grow up accepting these figures as the norm. For some, achieving that perfect body may be the natural result of eating well, exercising, and genetics. For others, such bodies never will be attainable. This breeds body dissatisfaction and an inability to measure up and fit in. The driven athlete, accustomed to hard work paying off, will try to attain that impossible body type, especially when they believe it will help their performance.

Boys aren't impervious to problems of body image. Five to 10 percent of those with eating disorders are boys or men, and this number might be increasing. Eating disorders in boys are most prevalent in sports that have weight classifications, such as wrestling and lightweight rowing or where a lighter body is perceived to be an advantage.

---

Jared had just turned 13 when his coach mentioned that he might be a faster runner if he lost his little belly. Jared was just beginning puberty and was naturally gaining weight even though he played soccer at a highly competitive level at least 10 hours a week.

The coach's comment was all Jared needed to channel his compliant spirit into developing a mild eating disorder. From that point on, Jared followed the pattern of dieters in his family. He cut out all sweets, limited his fats, and lost 10 pounds in three months. His family noticed quite soon that he wasn't eating, and although they initially complimented him on the weight loss, they noticed disturbing changes in his personality. But they had never heard about boys developing an eating disorder, so they did not immediately seek treatment. Soon Jared became too tired to play competitively. At that point, his family consulted his pediatrician, who referred him for nutrition counseling.

Fortunately, Jared was not in denial. Slowly, he added calories back, mainly in the form of higher-calorie beverages. Today, Jared plays Division I soccer. He realizes that his former coach had good intentions but probably should have never said anything about his weight gain.

---

Society accepts a wider range of male bodies, so boys are not subject to the same cultural pressures girls often feel to be unrealistically thin. Eating-disordered boys face other problems, though. Girls with eating disorders are sometimes envied by their peers for their adherence to restrictive diets and their resulting skinny bodies. Boys are often ostracized for their eating habits and the scrawny bodies that develop as a result of dieting. They are also less likely to be labeled as eating disordered because the disorders are relatively uncommon in boys. Consequently, they are less familiar with how to access treatment.

The typical eating-disordered behavior seen in male athletes tends to manifest itself in overexercising, purging, and dehydration rather than dietary restriction. Not everyone who relies on these dangerous methods develops an eating disorder, but the behaviors are unhealthy and dangerous and often lead to a lifetime of weight and eating struggles.

In addition to anorexia and bulimia, boys are also at risk for body dysmorphic disorder, a condition where one is obsessed with a real or imagined body flaw. They may be buff and built but see themselves as scrawny and thus develop a strong drive to achieve a muscular body. Ultimately, they are never satisfied with their bodies.

What makes athletes particularly vulnerable to eating disorders is that they often are the type of people who are driven to excel in an environment that may tolerate, even encourage, risky behavior in order to gain perceived benefits. Athletes are admired by their peers for their lean physiques, their healthy diets, and their self-discipline. They receive positive feedback from adults for their commitment. Their disorders may go undetected and their behaviors ignored because they are athletes—and this is sometimes part of their success.

## Start of a Problem

In some sports, a premium is placed on having a lighter, thinner body. A thinner body is a more capable body, athletes are told. This is certainly reinforced in our society. Studies show that from an early age, girls are more likely to befriend someone who is thin than someone who is overweight.

Most girls, regardless of the sport, want to be thin. All kids today are faced with enormous pressure to be thin in a country that is getting fatter. Waiflike bodies are idolized while super-size junk food is pervasive. Like all youths, those involved in sports are victims of this paradox.

In a country where childhood obesity is increasing dramatically, there are certainly kids participating in sports who would benefit from losing weight. But dieting or restricting food intake to lose weight to meet what might be an unrealistic goal can plant the seeds for unhappiness and a lifelong struggle with weight problems.

Dieting, warranted or not, is a precursor to developing an eating disorder. Not everyone who diets will develop an eating disorder, but anyone who has an eating disorder has dieted. Unfortunately, even an accurate assessment of a child's body weight and well-intentioned suggestion to lose a few pounds can have devastating consequences if delivered incorrectly or to a vulnerable child.

Coaches and parents don't cause eating disorders, but their well-intentioned comments can trigger problems in susceptible athletes. Coaches and parents need to be aware of how powerful their words are. A simple statement such as "If you lost a few pounds, you'd be faster" can be all it takes to send an eager-to-please but psychologically fragile athlete into an eating-disordered world (table 13.1).

Where does trouble lurk? One very delicate situation is for the prepubescent child who gains weight normally. At some point during normal growth and development, kids put on fat as they enter puberty. This weight gain is both noticeable and necessary. In our fat-phobic society, the additional weight might not be considered particularly attractive. Plus, weight gain can slow down a young athlete's performance.

**TABLE 13.1** What Coaches and Parents Should and Should Not Do

**What to do**

- The coach or trainer who has the best rapport with the person should arrange a private meeting. Never speak to the athlete about his or her eating behavior in the presence of another teammate.

- In an objective and nonpunitive way, list what you have seen and heard that has led you to be concerned. Let the athlete respond in full. Expect denial and rationalization.

- Emphasize that the person's place on the team or in the program will not be endangered by an admission of an eating disorder unless the eating disorder has compromised the person's health or put the athlete at risk for injury.

- If the athlete admits an eating disorder, try to determine if she or he can voluntarily abstain from the behaviors.

- If, in the face of compelling evidence, the athlete refuses to admit that a problem exists, or if it seems that the problem has either been longstanding or cannot be corrected readily, consult a clinician with expertise in treating eating disorders. If you work in a school athletic department, the school nurse or health center would be a good place to begin.

- Remember that most people with eating disorders have tried repeatedly and failed to correct the problem on their own. Failure is especially demoralizing to athletes who are always oriented toward success.

- Let the person know that eating disorders are treatable, and people do recover from them. Almost always, though, professional help is necessary. Needing help should not be regarded as a sign of weakness or inadequacy or lack of effort.

- Arrange for regular, private follow-up meetings apart from practice times.

- If the athlete is working with a physician or counselor, ask for permission to talk to that resource person.

- Remember that many athletes who develop eating disorders have been told that they need to lose weight. Realize that past or present coaches or trainers may have in some way contributed to the eating disorder. Let the athlete know that you are aware of the demands of the sport and how these demands may have played a role in the development of the problem.

(Continued)

**TABLE 13.1** Continued

**What not to do**

- Don't question teammates or talk to them about the athlete.
- If you have evidence that a problem exists, intervene. Don't hope it will go away if you ignore it.
- Don't tell the athlete that you know he or she has a problem without giving your reasons and evidence. This might make the athlete defensive.
- Don't tell the athlete to straighten up. Don't threaten to keep checking on him or her. He or she will feel increased stress that could make the eating disorder worse.
- Never conclude that if an athlete really wanted to stop the behaviors, he or she would. Don't make the mistake of believing that failure to improve shows a lack of effort. In this area, recovery can take years.
- Don't refuse to admit that you and the demands of the sport might have contributed to the problem.
- Don't try to keep the problem hidden by attempting to deal with it yourself when professional intervention is needed.
- Don't try to rescue the athlete single-handedly. These are complex problems that require professional intervention. Help the young athlete connect with professionals.

But prepubescent weight gain is important weight gain, needed to support an upcoming growth spurt. Because this weight gain is necessary and because this child is at that tender developmental stage where she (or he) might feel terribly uncomfortable with a changing body, to encourage this child to lose weight is entirely inappropriate and perhaps dangerous. This is not to suggest that weight loss is harmful or wrong or that children should never be encouraged to exercise more and eat less. But providing a child a diet that is too low in calories is never warranted. A healthy diet must meet the energy needs of an active, growing child. It must be a realistic plan and not overemphasize any one particular type of food or completely exclude a food group. For instance, most kids love junk foods. A healthy diet, even one for a child needing to lose weight, should include a reasonable amount of junk.

Cutting out junk and eating healthy might sound like sensible, helpful advice. Unfortunately, eating-disordered children, in their black and white world, misinterpret nutrition messages and blow them out of proportion. The perspective that some junk food is okay may escape an eating-disordered athlete.

## Consequences of Eating Disorders

There is never a good time to develop an eating disorder, but when a young athlete develops an eating disorder there can be profound and irreversible consequences. Restricting calories and nutrients during adolescence, when nutritional needs are the greatest, can retard puberty and permanently jeopardize growth.

The toll an eating disorder takes is not always immediate. Initially, many athletes manage to maintain a high level of training and performance. But eventually restriction, purging, or overexercising will leave the athlete malnourished and cause interference on many levels. Any athlete on a restrictive diet cannot maintain strength or training. Because of the restricted intake of important nutrients, eating-disordered athletes become more susceptible to illness. As starvation persists, their ability to concentrate wanes. This eventually impairs performance and puts them at risk for injury.

A serious consequence for the female eating-disordered athlete is the development of the female athlete triad. This condition results from restrictive eating, amenorrhea (lack of a menstrual period), and osteoporosis. The three are interrelated, but the general sequence is that the eating disorder causes the amenorrhea, and osteoporosis subsequently develops.

A female athlete can have any combination of the triad. In any case, the long-term consequences can be devastating. Left untreated, menstrual irregularities place the athlete at risk for fertility problems; osteoporosis can increase the risk for fractures and irreversible bone thinning.

Many female anorexic athletes are afraid to seek treatment for the problem. Treatment may mean modifying both their tendency to restrict food and to overexercise. They assume they'll hear, "You need to gain weight," which they believe means, "You need to get fat." These are the scariest words they can hear. And they are not true.

Treating an eating disorder is not just about eating more fat and gaining weight. To resume menstruation, the body needs more calories, more protein, and more fat. That might mean eventually weighing more, but there are some very thin girls who menstruate regularly.

Some of the consequences brought on by eating disorders are not always apparent. Although on the exterior an eating-disordered athlete may appear upbeat and happy, she is in fact totally preoccupied with food and weight. She is always hungry or thinking about how she is going to get rid of the food she has eaten. Those suffering are chronically crabby and moody from their insufficient food intake. Children with eating disorders withdraw socially. In a nutshell, someone with an eating disorder is paralyzed by obsessions about food, weight, exercise, and performance. Ultimately, they are miserable.

Sometimes eating disorders in athletes are disguised because it's easy to rationalize that athletes need to train hard, eat perfectly, and push their body to the limits. But training hard should not be confused with overexercise or compulsive activity. It can be difficult to differentiate training hard from overexercising or feeding the body healthfully from being obsessed with food.

But it isn't difficult to notice an athlete whose energy level is diminished, who is losing weight, and who is avoiding team meals. The bulimic athlete may not be as obvious as the athlete with anorexia. People with bulimia are often so ashamed and embarrassed about their problems that they become masters at covering it up. Concerned teammates frequently alert coaches and parents about the problems they see. Even if these concerned teammates seem to be dramatizing a situation, there's probably at least a grain of truth in what they're saying. Listen attentively and follow up on their concerns.

If a coach, parent, or teammate suspects an eating-disorder problem, it cannot be ignored. Although it's not the responsibility of coaches to provide therapy, they should make sure the problem is recognized and that treatment is sought. Unfortunately, eating disorders rarely just go away. The earlier the intervention, the greater the chance for successful treatment.

Once they recognize an eating disorder, coaches, parents, or concerned teammates need to approach the athlete delicately. The privacy of the athlete and his or her family must be respected. It's not unusual for an athlete to protest and try to minimize the reported problem. Denial is a hallmark of the disease. Unfortunately, some parents can be just as defensive when a problem is brought to their attention. However, most parents do what they can to help their child with the problem, which often involves seeking professional treatment.

A coach should not feel responsible for being a therapist, a nutritionist, or a doctor. Ideally, however, the treatment team of doctor, nutritionist, and therapist will also include the coach, because coaches can be extremely helpful in goal setting and motivation.

A coach plays a powerful role in the life of a young athlete and can be instrumental in treatment. Showing concern, addressing parents and teammates, and assuring athletes that their positions on the team aren't in jeopardy if they address the problem are all ways a coach can help the athlete.

The challenge in an appearance-based society is to prevent eating disorders before they start. This goal is complicated in the sports world because athletes often hear that the thinnest athlete is the best athlete. This view is then reinforced by society's love affair with emaciated media personalities. Coaches and parents should jump on every opportunity to promote the message that fitness is important, yes, but fitness is open to a much broader definition than being thin.

Young athletes are also absorbed by their self-image as athletes. They often can't separate the athlete from the rest of their identity. As a coach or parent, do your part by helping athletes feel secure in their abilities and letting these young, formative egos understand that they are much more than just the sports they play.

Eating disorders are a miserable way to live. The message to deliver loud and clear is that an eating-disordered athlete, regardless of what he or she weighs, is never a winner but is someone afflicted with a condition that must be dealt with and overcome.

---

## Sample Contract

Note: This is a contract between an athlete and a health care provider. Coaches should be aware of the details of this contract in order to support the athlete's goals.

To continue participating in sports and exercise programs, you must . . .

- eat and drink as instructed by your nutritionist
- gain a minimum of _____ pounds every two weeks or a total of _____ pounds a month.
  Starting weight today is _____ (range of _____)
- If weight loss occurs, you will withdraw from all activity until starting weight is regained and maintained for at least one week.
- If there is no weight gain over a two-week period, you must increase caloric intake by the prescribed amount and withdraw from activity until weight gain occurs.

Signed:

Athlete  _____

Parent  _____

Provider  _____

---

# Professional Resources

AED Academy for Eating Disorders
6728 Old McLean Village Dr., McLean, VA 22101
703-556-9222
www.aedweb.org

ANAD National Association of Anorexia Nervosa & Associated Disorders
P.O. Box 7, Highland Park, Il 60035
847-831-3438
www.ANAD.org

ANRED Anorexia Nervosa and Related Eating Disorders, Inc.
P.O. Box 5102, Eugene, OR 97405
503-344-1144
www.ANRED.com

Eating Disorder Referral and Information Center
2923 Sandy Pointe #6, Del Mar, CA 92014
858-792-7463
www.edreferral.com

Something Fishy Website on Eating Disorders
www.somethingfishy.org

## Talking to Your Athlete About Eating Disorders

- Eating disorders are serious problems that can result in death.
- Athletes may not experience problems with performance initially, but chronic undereating takes a toll on performance and ultimately on health and happiness.
- If a female athlete stops menstruating, she must bring this to the attention of her parents or physician.
- Coaches can help athletes feel comfortable at a weight that might not be ideal for a sport but that is ideal for the athlete.
- Eating disorders do not go away. They require medical attention to be resolved.

# Chapter 14

# CHAMPIONSHIP-WINNING RECIPES FOR YOUNG ATHLETES

As a working parent with two active children, my philosophy was that nothing should take more time to prepare than it does to eat. The recipes included here are basically food assembly: the art of combining nutritious ingredients in a few easy steps to satisfy simple taste buds without taxing the chef so much that he or she resents a picky eater for leaving a meal untouched.

The bulk of the recipes are a compilation of meals I have tested on my own family and with my clients and their families over the last 20 years. Others are recipes contributed by colleagues who prepare healthy meals for their families.

Feel free to improvise—use lean ground turkey in place of lean ground beef, turkey cutlets in place of chicken breast, tofu in place of cheese. Use more or fewer seasonings. To make a complete dinner, buy frozen vegetables and simply steam them and purchase salad greens and fruit prewashed and cut.

The portion sizes are approximate. You can easily double any recipe. All can be prepared and cooked ahead of time and reheated for late arrivals. After much thought, I chose not to include nutrient analyses for most recipes. I don't want people eating numbers. All of these recipes are nutritious, so don't worry about the calories and enjoy!

# Breakfast

Most young athletes don't take the time to eat a big breakfast. Many of these recipes take less than three minutes to prepare and can be eaten and enjoyed quickly. Athletes agree that they are a great way to start the day.

## Breakfast in a Cup

2 cups cereal such as Cheerios or Chex

1/4 cup craisins (dried cranberries) or raisins

2 tbsp peanuts or sunflower seeds

1. Mix together and store in an airtight container.
2. Stir into yogurt or eat as is.

Provided by Ann Chapman, RD.

## Peanut Butter Waffles

2 whole-grain frozen waffles

2 tbsp peanut butter

1 tbsp jam

1. Toast waffles.
2. Spread with peanut butter and jam.

Provided by Brenda Davy, PhD, RD, LD.

## Huevos Rancheros

1 corn tortilla

1 slice Monterey Jack cheese

1 whole egg

2 tbsp salsa

2 tbsp rice, beans or vegetables (optional)

Nonstick spray oil

1. Heat tortilla in microwave for 45 seconds.
2. Spray medium-sized skillet with nonstick spray oil.
3. Mix egg in a bowl with a fork and cook in heated pan until egg is no longer runny.
4. Place cheese on tortilla, cover with egg and salsa and optional toppings.
5. Roll up and cut in half to fit in plastic sandwich bag.

Provided by Marcia Greenblum MS, RD.

## Raisin Applesauce Muffins

1-1/2 cup unsweetened applesauce

1 large egg

2 tbsp oil

2 cups unbleached white flour

3/4 tsp baking soda

2 tsp baking powder

1/2 tsp cinnamon

3/4 cup raisins

Preheat oven to 375 degrees. Prepare muffin tins with paper liners.

1. Beat egg, oil, and applesauce in a large bowl.
2. Mix flour, baking soda, powder, and cinnamon in a bowl.
3. Add dry mixture to liquid and beat well.
4. Stir in raisins.
5. Spoon batter into muffin tins.
6. Bake 20 to 25 minutes. Cool on wire racks.

Makes 12 muffins

## English Muffin Sandwich

3 egg whites and 2 yolks

2 tbsp skim milk

1 tbsp butter or nonstick spray

1 sandwich-size English muffin

1 slice of muenster, cheddar, or Swiss cheese

1. Beat eggs and skim milk in small bowl.
2. Heat butter in small frying pan or spray with nonstick spray.
3. Toast English muffin in toaster.
4. Scramble eggs.
5. Spoon eggs onto muffin and top with cheese.

Serves 1

(Can be wrapped with foil and eaten in the car.)

## Meatless Main Dishes

These meatless dishes pack plenty of protein. Most can be prepared ahead of time and reheated as your hungry athlete walks in from practice.

### Baked Ziti

15 ounces low-fat ricotta cheese

8 ounces part-skim shredded mozzarella cheese

1 pound ziti

1 26-ounce or 32-ounce jar spaghetti sauce

2 tbsp grated parmesan cheese

1. Cook ziti as directed on box; drain well.
2. Combine ziti, ricotta, and mozzarella cheese.
3. Spread half of ziti mixture into bottom of a large casserole dish.
4. Pour one cup of sauce on top and sprinkle half the parmesan cheese over it.
5. Repeat this layer.
6. Cover with foil for oven or plastic wrap for microwave oven.
7. Conventional oven: Bake at 350 degrees for 25 minutes, remove foil, and continue baking another 15 minutes. Microwave: Cover with plastic wrap and cook 10 minutes. Uncover and heat another 5 minutes.

Serves 4 to 6

### Spinach Lasagna

2 10-ounce packages frozen, chopped spinach or 2 pounds fresh spinach

2 eggs, beaten

15 ounces low-fat ricotta cheese

1/2 tsp nutmeg

12 ounces lasagna noodles

4 cups tomato sauce

1-1/2 pounds shredded part-skim mozzarella cheese

*(continued)*

1. Cook spinach and drain well.
2. Mix cooked spinach with eggs, ricotta, and nutmeg.
3. Cook lasagna noodles (or use precooked noodles).
4. In a 9 × 13-inch baking dish, layer 1/3 cooked noodles, 1/2 spinach-cheese mixture, 1/3 sauce, and 1/3 mozzarella. Continue layering, ending with sauce and mozzarella.
5. Bake 45 minutes at 350 degrees. Let stand 10 minutes before cutting.

Serves 8 to 10

## Bean Burritos

4 flour tortillas
1 can refried beans
1/2 cup salsa
1/2 cup shredded cheddar cheese

1. Divide beans and spread on tortillas.
2. Top each tortilla with salsa and cheese.
3. Roll tortilla, tucking in at the end.
4. Heat on high for one minute in microwave to melt cheese.

Serves 4

## Black Beans and Rice Casserole

1-1/2 cups cooked rice
1 cup cooked black beans (canned are fine)
1-1/2 cups prepared salsa (reserve 1/4 cup)
1 cup low-fat shredded cheddar cheese (reserve 1/4 cup)

1. Spray baking dish with nonstick spray.
2. Combine all ingredients in baking dish.
3. Put reserved salsa and cheese on top.
4. Bake at 350 degrees about 20 minutes.

Serves 4

## Veggie Chili

2 tbsp oil

2 stalks celery, chopped

1 onion, chopped

1 green pepper, chopped

4 cloves garlic, minced

1 large can diced tomatoes

2 16-ounce cans red kidney beans, drained

1 16-ounce can whole kernel corn, drained

1 4-ounce can diced green chiles

1/4 cup chili powder

1 tbsp ground cumin

1. Heat oil in large pot. Add celery, onion, green pepper, and garlic; sauté until vegetables begin to soften (about 5 minutes).
2. Add all remaining ingredients. Bring to a boil.
3. Stir tomatoes with wooden spoon to break them up.
4. Reduce heat and simmer for 30 minutes, stirring occasionally.

Serves 4 to 6

## Peanut Butter Noodles

8 ounces uncooked pasta

4 scallions, chopped

1 cup cooked peas, chopped carrots, celery, peppers, or any combination of leftover cooked vegetables

1/4 cup peanut butter

1/4 cup soy sauce

1 tbsp oil

1/2 tsp garlic powder

1/4 tsp black pepper

1. Cook pasta as directed.
2. Blend peanut butter, soy sauce, oil, garlic powder, and black pepper.
3. Drain cooked pasta.
4. Pour sauce over pasta and mix well.
5. Add vegetables and serve.

Serves 4

### Beans With Pasta

1 can canillini beans, drained and rinsed

2 cups cooked penne or ziti

1 large bag frozen spinach, cooked and drained

salt and pepper to taste

1. Combine all ingredients in large pot.
2. Cook until heated through.

Serves 4

# Poultry and Meat

Chicken and turkey offer high-quality, lean protein. Boneless, skinless breasts cook quickly, so they're perfect for hungry athletes who can't wait until dinner. The following beef recipes use lean beef, which also prepares in a short time.

### Apricot Chicken

4 boneless, skinless chicken breasts

1/2 cup flour

1/4 tsp black pepper

Large resealable bag

Nonstick spray or 2 tbsp olive oil

1/2 cup apricot preserves

1 tbsp Dijon mustard

1/2 cup nonfat, plain yogurt

1. Preheat oven at 375 degrees.
2. Pour flour and pepper into plastic bag. Add chicken, reseal bag, and shake well until chicken is coated with flour.
3. Combine preserves, mustard, and yogurt in small bowl. Set aside.
4. Coat bottom of baking pan with spray or oil.
5. Place chicken in pan and bake 20 minutes.
6. Spread preserves mixture over chicken. Continue cooking 25 minutes.

Serves 4

## Barbecued Chicken Breasts

4 boneless, skinless chicken breasts

1/4 cup orange juice

1/2 cup prepared barbecue sauce

1/8 tsp black pepper

1/2 tbsp olive oil

1. Cut chicken breasts into long, narrow strips.
2. Combine orange juice, barbecue sauce, and black pepper.
3. Heat oil in frying pan.
4. Add chicken and stir-fry about 10 minutes or until chicken looks cooked.
5. Add sauce and heat to boil.

Serves 4

## Chicken Teriyaki

4 boneless, skinless chicken breasts, cut in small strips

3 tbsp pineapple juice

3 tbsp soy sauce

2 tbsp sherry

1 tbsp fresh ginger, grated

1/2 tsp dry mustard

2 cloves garlic, minced

1 tsp brown sugar

1. Combine all ingredients except chicken.
2. Place chicken in a baking pan. Pour marinade over it.
3. Cover and place in refrigerator at least an hour.
4. Grill or broil until done, turning often.

Serves 4

## East-West Chicken

8 pieces chicken (thighs, drumsticks, etc.)

2 tsp Dijon mustard

1/4 cup orange juice

1 tbsp olive oil

1/4 cup hoisin sauce

*(continued)*

1/4 cup chili sauce or barbecue sauce

pepper to taste

1. Place chicken in baking dish. Sprinkle with pepper.
2. In a small bowl, whisk orange juice into mustard.
3. Pour over chicken.
4. Combine hoisin sauce and chili sauce.
5. Bake chicken at 350 degrees 15 minutes.
6. Baste chicken with hoisin mixture. Continue baking about 20 minutes or place under broiler 10 minutes.

Serves 4

## Oven-Fried Chicken

4 boneless, skinless chicken breasts

1/4 cup skim milk

1/2 cup cornflake crumbs

1/4 cup grated parmesan cheese

salt and pepper to taste

2 tbsp olive oil or nonstick spray oil

1. Coat bottom of baking pan with spray or oil.
2. Combine crumbs and cheese in a bowl.
3. Season chicken breasts with salt and pepper.
4. Dip chicken into milk, then into crumb mixture.
5. Place chicken in dish. Bake at 350 degrees about 30 minutes, turning every 10 minutes.

Serves 4

## Turkey Burger

1-1/2 cups bread crumbs

1 tbsp olive oil

1-1/2 pounds ground turkey

Salt and pepper to taste

1. Combine all ingredients in bowl. Mix with hands until well blended.
2. Form into four patties.
3. Grill or broil 3 to 5 minutes per side.

Serves 4

## Fabulous Flank Steak

1-1/2 pound flank steak

1 large onion, sliced

1 cup mushrooms sliced

1/2 cup soy sauce

3 tbsp olive oil

Pepper

1. Sprinkle steak with pepper.
2. Put sliced onion and mushrooms over steak in a large, shallow baking dish.
3. Mix soy sauce and olive oil; pour over steak.
4. Cover with plastic wrap and refrigerate at least six hours.
5. Lift steak from marinade and broil about four minutes on each side.
6. While steak is broiling, pour marinade and vegetables into a small saucepan and heat to boil.
7. Let simmer 5 minutes.
8. When steak is done, slice on the diagonal and pour sauce over.

Serves 4

## Chili

1 tbsp olive oil

1 cup onion, chopped

1 carrot, chopped

1 cup green pepper, chopped

2 cloves garlic, minced

1-1/2 pounds ground beef

1 tbsp chili powder

1 tsp ground cumin

1/4 tsp cayenne pepper

1 28-ounce can tomatoes, drained and chopped

1 8-ounce can tomato sauce

1 can kidney beans, drained

*(continued)*

1. Sauté onions, carrot, pepper, and garlic in oil until onion is tender.
2. In a large pot, brown and drain meat.
3. Combine vegetables and all other ingredients except kidney beans.
4. Cook uncovered about 45 minutes.
5. Add beans. Simmer 10 more minutes.

Serves 4

## Quick Meatloaf

1/2 cup brown sugar

1 cup ketchup

2 tbsp Dijon mustard

1 tsp Worcestershire sauce

1 cup rolled oats

1/4 tsp black pepper

1 egg

1-1/2 pounds lean ground beef

1. Combine brown sugar, ketchup, mustard, and Worcestershire sauce in a medium bowl.
2. Mix oats, pepper, and egg in a large bowl.
3. Add half the brown sugar mixture to oats mixture; blend well.
4. Add ground beef and mix with your hands.
5. Pat mixture into loaf pan. Bake for an hour at 350 degrees.
6. Remove pan and pour remaining brown sugar mixture over meatloaf.
7. Bake an additional 15 minutes.

Serves 4 to 6

# Fish

Fish is the perfect fast food because it's healthy and rarely takes more than 15 minutes to prepare. Ounce for ounce, fish is about as pure a protein as you can get. Many people steer clear of fish because they don't know how to buy it or prepare it. To make friends with fish, start by buying the freshest fish available from a reputable market. Choose a marinade or topping with familiar ingredients.

## Baked Fish Tenders

1-1/2 pounds flounder, tilapia, perch, or other white fillet

3/4 cup skim milk

1/2 tsp dried mustard

1/4 tsp pepper

1/2 cup bread crumbs

1 lemon

2 tbsp oil or nonstick spray oil

1. Coat bottom of baking pan with spray or oil.
2. Combine bread crumbs, pepper, and mustard in small bowl.
3. Dip fish in milk and then in bread crumb mixture.
4. Place in greased dish and squirt lemon over fish.
5. Bake at 350 degrees 8 to 10 minutes.

Serves 4

## Fish Kabobs

1 pound swordfish, tuna, or other firm fish cut in 1-inch cubes

1/4 cup pineapple juice

2 tbsp soy sauce

2 tbsp sherry

1 tsp brown sugar

1/2 tsp dried mustard

1 clove garlic, minced

1 tsp grated ginger

2 tbsp oil

1. Combine all ingredients except fish.
2. Place fish in pan, cover with marinade, and place in refrigerator for at least an hour.

*(continued)*

3. Using skewers, make kabobs. Add vegetables and fruit as desired.
4. Broil about 10 to 12 minutes, turning once.

Serves 4

## Company Poached Fish

1-1/2 pounds salmon, orange roughy, or other filet

1 red pepper, cut in strips

1/2 onion, chopped

6 sliced mushrooms

1 tbsp lemon juice

1/4 tsp garlic powder or 1 garlic clove, minced

2 tbsp soy sauce

1 tbsp olive oil

Foil

1. Place each fish filet on a square piece of foil, large enough to cover the fish.
2. Divide vegetables over each fish filet.
3. In a small bowl, combine lemon juice, soy sauce, garlic, and olive oil. Pour it evenly over filets.
4. Close foil around filet.
5. Bake in oven at 350 degrees about 20 minutes.

Serves 4

## Easy Cajun Fish Filets

1-1/2 pounds tilapia, flounder, perch, or other white filets

1 lemon

2 tbsp Old Bay seasoning

2 tbsp oil or nonstick spray oil

1. Coat bottom of baking pan with spray or oil.
2. Place fish in baking dish.
3. Squirt lemon over fish.
4. Sprinkle seasoning over fish.
5. Bake at 350 for 12 minutes.

Serves 4

## Honey Mustard Fish

1-1/2 pounds firm fish filet such as salmon, swordfish, or grouper

Olive oil

1 lemon

4 tbsp Dijon mustard

2 tbsp honey

1. Brush filets with olive oil.
2. Squirt lemon over fish.
3. Combine honey and mustard.
4. Paint fish with honey mixture.
5. Broil fish about 15 to 20 minutes, depending on thickness of fish.

Serves 4

## Fish Marinade

This will make enough to marinade 1-1/2 pounds to 2 pounds of fish.

3 tbsp soy sauce

3 tbsp lemon juice

3 tbsp sugar

2 tbsp olive oil

Combine all ingredients.

## Shrimp or Scallop Stir Fry

1 8-ounce can sliced water chestnuts

1 large red pepper, cut into thin strips

2 green onions, cut into thin slices

1 package frozen, stir-fry vegetables

2 tbsp olive oil

2 tsp cornstarch

1 tsp sugar

1/4 tsp ground ginger

3/4 cup chicken broth

2 tbsp soy sauce

1 tbsp rice vinegar

*(continued)*

1 pound peeled shrimp

1 pound scallops

1. Combine cornstarch, sugar, ginger, broth, soy sauce, and vinegar in a small bowl.
2. Heat oil in frying pan. Add onions, pepper, and frozen vegetables and cook until soft.
3. Add fish and stir-fry until cooked, about 5 minutes.
4. Pour in liquid mixture. Heat through.

Serves 4

# Pizza and Wraps

Pizza and wraps are the perfect vehicle for topping with nutritious ingredients. Add a salad or soup and a glass of milk and you can have an easy, healthy meal.

## Pizza

If you don't have time to make pizza dough, use premade crust or French bread for this pizza recipe.

15-ounce jar pizza sauce

1-1/2 cups shredded low-fat mozzarella cheese

2 tbsp olive oil

Optional toppings: green peppers, sliced olives, cooked hamburger, tuna, leftover vegetables

1. Cover a baking sheet with foil. Lay crust on baking sheet. If using French bread, cut the bread in half, top to bottom. Then slice each half again so that you have four long pieces.
2. Drizzle oil over crust or bread. Then spread with pizza sauce.
3. Sprinkle with cheese. Top with any desired topping.
4. Broil 8 to 10 minutes until cheese begins to bubble.

Serves 4

## Veggie Wraps

4 flour tortillas

1/2 cup humus

1 cup lettuce, shredded

1/2 cucumber, peeled and chopped

1. Moisten tortillas with a few drops of water. Cover with a paper towel and heat in the microwave 45 seconds.
2. Divide humus over each tortilla.
3. Top with vegetables.
4. Roll up tortilla.

Serves 4

## Peanut Butter and Apple Wrap

4 flour tortillas

8 tbsp peanut butter

1 apple, peeled and chopped

1. Moisten tortillas with a few drops of water. Cover with a paper towel and heat in the microwave 45 seconds.
2. Spread each tortilla with 2 tbsp peanut butter.
3. Sprinkle apple over each tortilla.
4. Roll up tortilla.

Serves 4

## Perfect Pita Pockets

2 whole wheat pita breads

1 cup egg salad, tuna salad, or chicken salad

Lettuce, tomato, water chestnuts

1. Carefully cut opening in pita.
2. Fill each pita with half cup of salad.
3. Top with vegetables.

## Individual Quesadillas

4 fajita-size flour tortillas

4 tsp butter or margarine

1 cup shredded cheese

4 tbsp salsa

1. Spread butter or margarine over tortilla.
2. Heat frying pan.
3. Place one tortilla in pan, butter side down.
4. Sprinkle with cheese.
5. Add next tortilla, buttered side up, on top of cheese.
6. Sprinkle with cheese.
7. Continue stacking next two tortillas. Cook until cheese begins to melt.
8. Remove from pan. Cut into four wedges. Top each wedge with salsa and serve.

Serves 4

# Beverages

For times when your young athlete would rather drink a meal than sit down and eat, here are some tasty, nutritious options.

Directions for building a better smoothie:

1. Put frozen ingredients in the blender first. Make sure they're no larger than golf ball size.
2. Add liquid next.
3. Blend briefly, then add fruit and other ingredients.
4. Add more liquid if needed.

## Protein-Plus Smoothie

Substitute blended, nonfat yogurt and skim milk to reduce calories.

1 cup frozen fruit

1 cup yogurt

1 tbsp protein powder or packet of protein powder

1 cup 2-percent milk

1 cup fruit juice

Blend all ingredients in blender.

## Coffee-Flavored Breakfast Smoothie

Substitute nonfat yogurt and skim milk to reduce calories.

1 cup coffee-flavored yogurt

1 cup 2-percent milk

1 envelope instant breakfast

1 banana, sliced in pieces

2 tbsp peanut butter

10 to 12 ice cubes

   Blend all ingredients in blender.

## Vegan Smoothie

1 cup vanilla soy beverage

1-1/2 ounces cubed tofu

1 banana

1/2 tsp vanilla

1 tbsp honey or sugar

10 ice cubes

   Blend all ingredients in blender.

## Homemade Sports Drink

4 tbsp sugar

1/4 tsp salt

1/4 cup hot water

1/4 cup orange juice (not concentrate) or 2 tbsp lemon juice

3-3/4 cups cold water

1. In the bottom of a pitcher, dissolve the sugar and salt in the hot water.

2. Add juice and remaining water; chill.

Makes 1 quart.

From *Nancy Clark's Sports Nutrition Guidebook*, 2003, Human Kinetics Publishing.

# Snacks and Desserts

We eat desserts because they taste good and don't necessarily have to be nutritious. The desserts and snacks listed here do have some nutritional value—but they still taste good!

## Baked Apple

4 large baking apples

1/2 cup dried cranberries or golden raisins

1/4 cup light brown sugar

2 tsp butter

1/3 cup apple juice or cider

1. Using a vegetable peeler, remove a thin slice from the bottom of each apple so it will stand. Remove a 1/2-inch slice from the top of each apple. With a melon baller or grapefruit spoon, scoop out center core of each apple, leaving bottom intact.
2. Stir cranberries or raisins and brown sugar together in a small bowl.
3. Spoon 1/4 of mixture into apple cavity.
4. Place apples in small baking dish. Dot each apple with 1/2 tsp butter.
5. Pour juice or cider around apples and cover dish tightly with foil.
6. Bake 30 minutes at 450 degrees. Uncover and baste apples with the juice; bake 10 more minutes, basting a few more times.

Serves 4

## Apple Crisp

4 cups baking apples

1/2 cup unbleached white flour

1/2 cup rolled oats

3/4 cup brown sugar

3/4 tsp ground nutmeg

3/4 tsp ground cinnamon

dash salt

1/3 cup butter                                            *(continued)*

1. Peel and slice apples; place in greased 8 × 8-inch pan.
2. Mix flour, oats, sugar, nutmeg, cinnamon, and salt.
3. Cut in the butter.
4. Spread mixture over apples.
5. Bake at 375 degrees for 30 minutes.

Serves 8

## Apricot Raspberry Whip

1/2 cup dried apricots

1/2 cup orange juice

1/4 cup sugar

1-1/2 cups vanilla yogurt

1/2 cup fresh or frozen raspberries, thawed

1. In medium saucepan, combine apricots, juice, and sugar.
2. Bring to a boil. Reduce heat and simmer until apricots are tender (about 10 minutes).
3. Mix yogurt and apricots together. Chill at least one hour. Top with raspberries.

Serves 4

## Fruit Kabobs With Dip

Fresh fruit such as cantaloupe, honeydew, watermelon balls, chunks of peaches or pineapple, orange sections, grapes

Kabob sticks or toothpicks

1. Wash and dry fruit.
2. Thread on stick.
3. Use dip (recipe following) if desired.

## Quick Yogurt Dip for Fruit

1 6-ounce container of vanilla yogurt *or* 1 cup unsweetened applesauce

1 cup plain yogurt

1 tsp ground cinnamon

1. Blend applesauce and yogurt together.
2. Sprinkle with cinnamon.

## Quick Yogurt-Mustard Dip for Vegetables

1 cup plain yogurt

3 tbsp Dijon mustard

Sprinkle of dill

Combine all ingredients.

## Yogurt/Spinach Dip for Vegetables

1 10-ounce package frozen spinach

1 cup plain yogurt

1/4 cup light mayonnaise

2 tbsp grated parmesan cheese

1. Cook spinach as directed. Drain and squeeze out excess liquid.
2. Combine all ingredients with spinach.
3. Cool before serving.

## Apple Bagel Sandwich

1/2 bagel

1 slice of cheese

1/2 green apple, sliced

Cinnamon

1. Place cheese slice on bagel half.
2. Top with apple. Sprinkle with cinnamon.
3. Put in 350-degree oven 5 to 10 minutes or until cheese starts to melt.

Serves 1

## Mock Crepe

1 8-inch flour tortilla

1/4 cup cottage cheese

2 tbsp applesauce

Dash of cinnamon

1. To soften tortilla, drizzle warm water on tortilla and place in microwave for 10 seconds.

*(continued)*

2. Mix cottage cheese, applesauce, and cinnamon in a small bowl.
3. Spread mixture over warmed tortilla.
4. Roll tortilla with mixture on inside.
5. Heat in microwave about 30 seconds.

Serves 1

## Homemade Ice Cream Sandwich

2 graham crackers

1/4 cup frozen yogurt or ice cream

1. Spread ice cream on one graham cracker.
2. Place other graham cracker on top.

Serves 1

# Index

NOTE: The italicized *f* and *t* following page numbers refer to figures and tables, respectively. The italicized *ff* and *tt* following page numbers refer to multiple figures and tables, respectively.

## A

## B

# C

# D

Davy, Brenda  146
dehydration. *See also* fluids
    effects of  24–25
    signs of  24*t*, 27
designer waters  124
DHEA  122–123
*Diagnostic and Statistical Manual of Mental Disorders (DSM)*  133
dietary fat  48
Dietary Guidelines for Americans  61*f*
dietary reference intakes (DRI)  12, 13*t*–16*t*
dietary supplements  55
dieting
    healthy weight ranges  60–62, 60*f*
    parental reinforcement  67–68
    proper weight loss  49
    weight gain  55–57, 56*t*, 57*tt*
diets. *See also* specific sports
    cooking thin guidelines  70
    the eat more diet  56*t*
    evaluating programs  67
    modified lacto-ovo vegetarian  37
    modified vegetarian  40
*Diets Designed for Athletes*  104*t*
dinner, five-day rotation  99, 100*t*. *See also* recipes
diuretics  28
diving  92–93
DRI (dietary reference intakes)  12, 13*t*–16*t*

# E

eating disorders. *See* specific disorders, such as bulimia
    about  133
    at-risk athletes  136
    and body image  137
    consequences of  140–143
    professional resources  143–144
    triggers for  138–139, 139*t*–140*t*
the eat more diet  56*t*
ectomorphs  51–52, 52*f*
electrolytes  27–28
elements. *See* minerals
empty calories  8–9
endomorphs  51–52, 52*f*

# S

salad bars  111, 112*t*–113*t*
self-esteem
    and body changes  4–5, 59
    parents and coaches role in  5
self-image  62–63
sensible snacking  101
shaving calories  66*t*
simple carbohydrates  8, 43
sleep, and energy levels  5–6, 6*t*
snack foods  69*t*
snacking
    at games  131
    sensible  101
snacks  99
soccer  80–82
softball  74–75
somatotypes  51–52, 52*f*
spirit bags  20
sports. *See* specific events
sports bars, comparing  104*t*
sports bars, with lycopene  124
sports drinks  27–28, 118
standard height and weight chart  60*f*
starch  44
Subway menu options  114*t*
super-size meals  110–111
supplements
    dietary  55
    ergogenic  117–118
    mineral  8
    protein  35–36
    quality control  119–120, 120*t*
    vitamin  8
sweating
    conditions affecting  23–24
    replacing electrolytes  27–28
swimming  84–86

# T

Taco Bell menu options  114*t*
talking to your athlete about
    carbohydrates  50
    dietary needs for their sport  96

# U

# V

# W

## Z

# About the Author

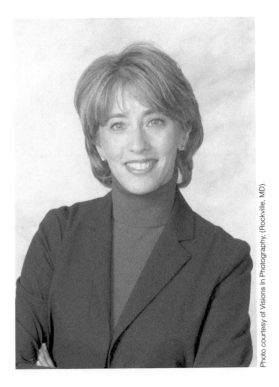

Photo courtesy of Visions In Photography, (Rockville, MD).

**Ann Litt,** MS, RD, LD, who passed away in 2007, was a nutrition expert who had been in private practice since 1980 and consulted many athletes and their parents on proper nutritional practices. She specialized in helping teenagers and young adults develop normal eating habits. In addition, she was a nutrition consultant to the Washington Redskins and the Elite Athlete Training System (EATS).

Litt is the author of *The College Student's Guide to Eating Well on Campus* and was highly regarded among nutritionists and conducted workshops nationwide.

She was a chairperson of Nutrition Entrepreneurs, a dietetic practice group of the American Dietetic Association (ADA), and was the recipient of the Recognized Young Dietitian Award from the ADA.

Litt lived outside Washington, DC; she is survived by her husband and two sons.

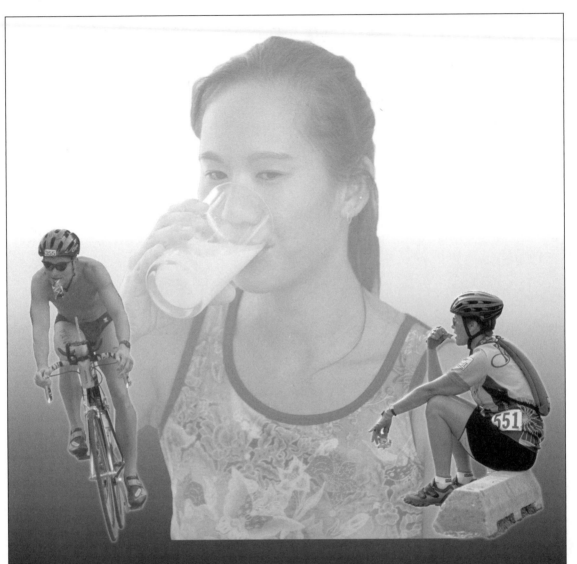

You'll find other outstanding sports nutrition resources at

**www.HumanKinetics.com/nutritioninsport**

In the U.S. call 1-800-747-4457

Australia 08 8372 0999 • Canada 1-800-465-7301
Europe +44 (0) 113 255 5665 • New Zealand 0800 222 062

 **HUMAN KINETICS**
*The Premier Publisher for Sports & Fitness*
P.O. Box 5076 • Champaign, IL 61825-5076 USA